History of Healthcare Policy in Republic of Korea

Myongsei SOHN · So Yoon Kim
Representative Author

Yunhong Noh · Dong-hyun LEE · Sunjoo Kang
Yuri Lee · Sang Sook Beck · Siwoo Kim · Hyojung Sea
Co-Author

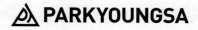

History of Healthcare Policy in Republic of Korea

Printed the first edition in 2023. 11. 24
Published the first edition in 2023. 12. 7

Representative Author   Myongsei SOHN · So Yoon Kim

President   Jong-Man An · Sang-Joon An
Publishing Company   Parkyoung Publishing & Company
                        #210, 53, Gasan digital 2-ro, Geumcheon-gu, Seoul
                        Registered in 1959.3.11. 300-1959-1

tel   82-2-733-6771
fax   82-2-736-4818
e-mail   pys@pybook.co.kr
homepage   www.pybook.co.kr

ISBN 979-11-303-1770-0   93510

A special acknowledgement to the National Research Foundation of Korea(NRF) who supported the capacity building
project between Yonsei and UHAS, as well as the production of this book.
(No.2021H1A7A2A03098782 / Public Health Educational Capacity Development of University of Health and Allied Sciences
in Ghana.)

19,000 ₩ (Korean Currency)

Preface

We are very delighted that the book "History of Healthcare Policy in Republic of Korea" is going to be published.

This book provides information on the history and development process of Korea's healthcare policy and the transformation process of the healthcare system. The vast amount of research data collected in this book is believed to be a major foundation for the development of the healthcare system and conducting research on policies in the future. In addition, We believe that this book can be an important resource tool for establishing healthcare projects and policies in developing countries.

The 2019 World Health Assembly adopted an ambitious resolution recognizing the role of healthcare system and policy in providing the full range of health services needed throughout the life course, including prevention, treatment, rehabilitation, and palliative care. Achieving the health-related SDGs, including UHC, will not be possible without a stronger healthcare system and policy.

The current healthcare system in Korea is the product of continuous development over the history of 80 years. Although the system is not in the ultimate, finalized state but still in the process of improvement in all dimensions, the Korean healthcare system has achieved a high level of development compared to that of advanced countries in terms of the health of national population or industrialization. However, this high level of healthcare system is not something that has been achieved by an overnight miracle or by simple adoption of other countries' systems. The healthcare system as an institution is a historical product of continuous development in which all related parties in healthcare - health professionals, those responsible for drafting and enforcement of health policy, and the general public - are involved in shaping and changing the system to suit specific situations of Korea in the midst of turbulent changes that the society has experienced since the enlightenment period of the country. In this context, there is no doubt that the domestic healthcare system is currently in a highly mature stage, but it is also evident that there are still a range of problems that need to be addressed and resolved. In order to identify these problems, it is necessary to examine and study the historical background from an objective standpoint, draw implications for today's healthcare system in Korea, and come up with rational solutions for real−world problems based on the lessons learned from the history. This will serve as a sensible and articulate basis for establishing the future direction and targets of the healthcare system in Korea.

In this book, the records from 1959 to 2020 related to governmental projects, policies, and institutions held by the government or healthcare—related organizations that are judged to have value in health history are investigated and objective accounts on the records and data are described. Thus, the healthcare policy and system have been described as "actions and products that are performed or produced for adequate combination of the state intervention and the principles of market economy for fair distribution of health and medical resources under the principle of equity and efficiency with a view to promoting public health and satisfying the demand for treatment of diseases". Based on the definition and general perception, the content of this book is divided into three categories as follows. First, the overall public healthcare system in Korea has been reviewed. Second, in terms of healthcare policies implemented under this system, data and materials on health insurance, separation of dispensary from medical practice and healthcare industry have been reviewed. Third, data and materials on management of infectious disease in terms of prevention and disease management have been reviewed. However, all policies, projects, and institutions were not planned or implemented as a single, isolated policy or project, and all of these were executed or implemented in an organic and interdependent relationship. Therefore, Chapters 2 and 3 provide detailed information on the respective aspect, but in order to understand the relationship between these contents in a broader framework, it would be helpful to look into the overall historical flow from the viewpoint of healthcare policy considering the time of the milestone events in understanding the changes in healthcare system in Korea. In this context, this book provides an account on various projects, policies and institutions related to healthcare system of Korea in light of the change of the times with historical perspectives.

In order to share these valuable experiences and cases of healthcare policy in the international community, we are publishing an English of healthcare policy history.

This work is part of the Health and Medical Education Competency Enhancement Project of the University of Health & Allied Science (UHAS) in Ghana, which is facilitated by the Ministry of Education and supported by the National Research Foundation (NRF) of Korea.

The goal of this project is to make the UHAS experience a new leap forward as a health—specialized higher education institution in Ghana while strengthening the capabilities of community health education at UHAS's medical school, nursing school, and health school.

The aim is to help UHAS cultivate differentiated healthcare professionals in the health sector who can then help improve the health standards in Ghana and other countries in Africa.

Therefore, we are preparing to provide a practical reference textbook that can provide information on building, changing, and implementing healthcare's strategies so that professors and students can appropriately apply them in the field of healthcare in each stage of economic growth.

Further, we hope that this book will help establish realistic, affordable, and effective healthcare delivery systems and policy that are tailored to the economic and cultural level of each developing communities that still lack access to essential services for healthcare policy.

We sincerely appreciate the co – authors, editorial board members, researchers for helping us with this tedious and continuous work. We would like to thank to Dr. Yunhong Noh, Prof. Dong-hyun LEE, Prof. Sunjoo Kang, Prof. Yuri Lee, Prof. Sangsook Beck, and Dr. Siwoo Kim and the researchers, Ms. Hyojung Sea(saina), Ms. Dasol Jessica Ro and Ms. Jiwon Park for their invaluable assistance in participating in the project and helping write and edit this book. We also appreciate professional proofreading given by Editage.

Lastly, we would like to express our gratitude to the researchers who made efforts to publish this book while participating in the project, as well as the National Research Foundation of Korea(NRF) who supported the production of this book. We would also like to thank Parkyoung Publishing & Company for their guidance throughout this publishing process.

Dr. Myongsei SOHN
Chairman, RIGHT Fund
Former President, HIRA
Emeritus Professor, Yonsei University

Prof. So Yoon Kim
Yonsei University College of Medicine
Director, Asian Institute for Bioethics and Health Law

About the Representative Authors

Myongsei SOHN

MD, MPH, PhD, is a Chairman of RIGHT Fund and Executive Council member of Council for International Organization of Medical Sciences (CIOMS).
Now, he is working as a Executive Director, Institute for Global Engagement & Empowerment(IGEE), Yonsei University and Emeritus Professor of Department of Preventive Medicine and Public Health, Yonsei University College of Medicine in Korea. And he is Former President of Health Insurance Review and Assessment Service (HIRA) and Asia Pacific Academic Consortium for Public Health (APACPH). Also, he is Former Vice Chairperson of Executive Board for World Health Organization (WHO) and Former Member of International Bioethics Committee for United Nations Educational, Scientific and Cultural Organization (UNESCO).

So Yoon Kim

MD, MPH, PhD, is a Professor of Division of Medical Law and Ethics, Department of Humanities and Social Medicine, Yonsei University College of Medicine in Korea.
Now, she is working as a director of the Asian Institute for Bioethics and Health Law (WHO Collaborating Center for Health Law & Bioethics) and Division of International Health Science, Graduate School of Public Health, Yonsei University. And she is President of Korean Association of Medical Law and Asia Pacific Academic Consortium for Public Health (APACPH). Also, she is serving as editor−in−chief of the Journal of Global Health Science (JGHS) in the Korean Society of Global Health.

About the Co-Author Members

Yunhong Noh

PhD, is a Chairman of Korea Pharmaceutical and Bio—Pharma Manufacturers Association (KPBMA). He served as a Senior secretary to the President for employment and welfare and Commisioner of Korea Food and Drug Administration (KFDA).

Dong-hyun LEE

PhD. in public health. His PhD. thesis is "Improvement of Payment System for Chronic Disease Management; A Comparative and institutional study on the Case of USA and Japan." He is a research professor at the Department of Global Health Science, the School of Public Health, Yonsei University. He majored in Health Administration at Yonsei University. His research interest is Global Health Science, Public Health Policy, Public Health Education and Quality Improvement of Health care Service Payment System.

Sunjoo Kang

PhD. in Law and Nursing, is a research professor at the Graduate School of Public Health, Yonsei University. With 13 years of experience as a nursing faculty member, she joined the university in 2019. She served as a nursing officer in the Korean Army and has actively participated in diverse global health projects since 2012. Sunjoo is an associate editor for the Frontiers in Public Health Journal and is recognized as a global nursing leader trained by the International Council of Nurses.

Yuri Lee

RN, MPH, MSc, PhD, is an Assistant Professor at the Department of Health and Medical Information at Myongji College in Korea. She has served as the Director of General Affairs of the Korean Society of Global Health. Also, she is a member of the Editorial Board of the Journal of Global Health Science.

Sang Sook Beck

MPH, PhD, is a Research Professor at the Graduate School of Public Health, Yonsei University in Korea. She also works as Secretary General of the Korea Golden Age Forum.

Siwoo Kim

RDH, PhD, is a senior researcher at SNU Medical Research Center, Institute of Environmental Medicine, Seoul National University in Korea. She studied in Yonsei University and participated in various ODA (Official Development Assistance) projects related to health.

Hyojung Sea (saina)

RN, MPH, is a Researcher of Asian Institute for Bioethics and Health Law of Yonsei University (WHO Collaborating Centre for Health Law & Bioethics) and Doctoral Program in Medical Law and Ethics, Yonsei University. She is a nurse with over 17 years of clinical experience, served as the team leader of the Slioam International Center for the Disabled People and participated the ODA projects such as international development cooperation, global health, and for international disabled.

About the Editorial Board

* Editor-In-Chief : So Yoon Kim

MD, MPH, PhD, is a Professor of Division of Medical Law and Ethics, Department of Humanities and Social Medicine, Yonsei University College of Medicine in Korea.
Now, she is working as a director of the Asian Institute for Bioethics and Health Law (WHO Collaborating Center for Health Law & Bioethics) and Division of International Health Science, Graduate School of Public Health, Yonsei University. And she is President of Korean Association of Medical Law and Asia Pacific Academic Consortium for Public Health (APACPH). Also, she is serving as editor－in－chief of the Journal of Global Health Science (JGHS) in the Korean Society of Global Health.

* Editorial Board Member

Yumi SON

MPH, is a Researcher of Asian Institute for Bioethics and Health Law of Yonsei University (WHO Collaborating Centre for Health Law & Bioethics) and Doctoral Program in Medical Law and Ethics, Yonsei University.

Jong Hyuk Lee

Consultant, World Health Organization Regional Office for the Western Pacific.

Dasol Jessica Ro

MBA, ia a Researcher of Asian Institute for Bioethics and Health Law of Yonsei University (WHO Collaborating Centre for Health Law & Bioethics) and Doctoral Program in Medical Law and Ethics, Yonsei University.

Contents

Preface   iii

Chapter 1.

Overview of History of Healthcare Policy in Korea

Section 1. Before 1945; Historical Background of Healthcare Policy   3

Section 2. From 1945 to 1960s; Birth of Healthcare Policy   9

Section 3. From 1970s to 1980s; Expanding Healthcare Policies   13

Section 4. From 1990s to 2000s; Ongoing Efforts to Improve the Quality of Life for the Public   19

Chapter 2.

Changes in policies for providing medical services in Korea

Section 1. Establishment of Public Health System   29

Section 2. Current Status and Future Development of Healthcare Resources   35

Section 3. Changes in Health Care Organizations and the Present   45

Section 4. Aspects of the Development of Changes in the Health Insurance System   57

Section 5. Changes in Drugs and the Pharmaceutical Industry   65

Section 6. Changes in Health Promotion Policies   81

Section 7. Promotion of Maternal and Child Health and Implementation of Family Planning   89

Section 8. Changes in Policies for Disease Control and Eradication   101

Chapter 3.

Discussion of major issues with respect to changes in healthcare policy

Section 1. Beginning of the Debate on Bioethics and Safety
and the Transition Process   115

Section 2. Discussion on the institution of induced abortion   125

Section 3. Attempts to Introduce For-Profit Medical Corporations   135

Section 4. Conflicts of Various Issues Following Separation of
Prescribing and Dispending   147

Section 5. Traditional Korean Medicine Policy and Conflict between
Traditional Korean Medicine Doctors and Pharmacists   161

Section 6. Response to New Infectious Diseases and Public
Health Crisis   173

Reference   193

Table

〈Table 1〉 Annual Trends of Public Health Centers and Community
          Health Posts   30

〈Table 2〉 Maternal and child health projects by life cycle   98

〈Table 3〉 Main areas of debate on inclusion in the Bioethics Act   118

〈Table 4〉 Types of medical corporation   138

〈Table 5〉 Comparison between for-profit and nonprofit medical
          corporations   139

Figure

〈Figure 1〉 Health Care System from Medical Insurance Act   16

〈Figure 2〉 Development objectives of Korea's health industry
           in stages   21

〈Figure 3〉 Number of outpatients visits per capita (2018)   22

〈Figure 4〉 Public Health Delivery System   31

〈Figure 5〉 Medical insurance system (July 1977 - November 1998)   60

〈Figure 6〉 The first Western-style hospital, Jejungwon   66

Chapter 1

Overview of History of Healthcare Policy in Korea

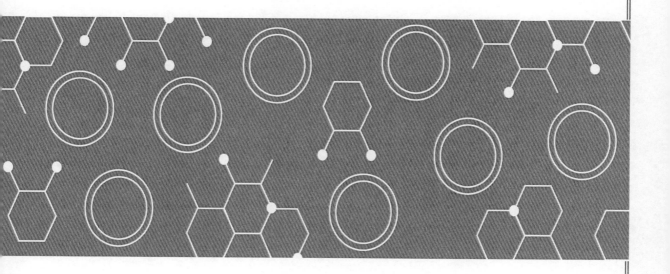

Section 1
Before 1945; Historical Background of Healthcare Policy

1. Introduction of Western medicine

The shaping of the healthcare system of Korea during the Joseon Dynasty and Japanese colonial period started with the introduction of Western medicine, which led to official recognition of Western medicine doctors and their settlement within the existing system of traditional medicine providers. If Joseon at the time had been a stable society with established systems, when a new system of modern doctors' license was introduced in the conventional system of traditional medicine, it would have led to fierce opposition, making it tremendously difficult to accept the transition into the new concept and system of doctors' license. However, at the end of the Joseon Dynasty in 1884, Min Young—ik, the nephew of Empress Myeongseong, who was seriously wounded by an assassin's knife during the Ujeongguk Incident, experienced dramatic recovery of his condition thanks to the surgical treatment of Horace N. Allen (安連), who was a doctor at the US legation residing in Joseon at that time. Therefore, Dr. Allen gained the trust of Emperor Gojong, the ruler of Joseon, and became the court physician without going through public policy discussion, which led to the introduction of Western medicine doctors to the orthodox health system of the country. Under usual circumstances, this process would have led to internal debates, which may cause social division and conflict, but backed by the determination and active support of Gojong, the first hospital of Korea opened in an abandoned house of Hong Young—Sik in Jae—dong, Seoul on April 10, 1885. Two days after the opening, the hospital was given the official name Gwanghyewon (廣惠院: House of Extended Grace), the first modern medical institution in Joseon, but was renamed Chejungwon (濟衆院: Widespread Relief House) a few days later. Since the Gapsin Coup in 1884, Dr. Allen experienced difficulties of having no proper treatment facility for patient treatment, and in order to resolve the problem, he proposed a plan to build a national hospital to the government of Joseon in January 1885. The proposed hospital plan stated that the treatment for patients and medical education can be conducted in the hospital, and since the government of Joseon also appreciated the necessity of introduction of Western medicine, the proposal was accepted, leading to the official recognition of Western medicine and acquisition of treatment rights of Western medicine doctors in Joseon. This was a drastic and revolutionary change that could even be described as a bloodless coup. In the midst of extreme social chaos, accepting the Western medicine system with the highest efficacy and obtaining the rights of treatment for Western medicine doctors were possible without having to undergo unnecessary debates. Indeed, for introduction of a new system and its settlement and stabilization, there was a problem of mobilizing financial resources such as government budget allocation and utilization of resources of private sector. However, for treatment of the conservative society on the whole, traditional medicine was practiced, and foreign loan and aid were used for financial resources and gradually Western medicine has introduced into the mainstream of Joseon society.

After Dr. Allen, Drs Heron (惠論, John W. Heron) and Avison (魚丕信, Oliver R. Avison), Western medicine doctors in the United States, Canada, and Europe, played a central role in establishing modern medicine in Joseon. They raised funds through the government, religious foundations, and charitable organizations to finance the establishment of the modern hospital in Joseon society. Through their efforts, the usefullness and effect of modern medicine was recognized in Korea, and the next generation of doctors for medical practice for Koreans was nurtured, who led the operation of the hospitals and medical research. A number of different stories have passed down from different perspectives, and deep－rooted debate on modern medicine has continued to the present day. The historical significance of this period is that it has greatly contributed to the development of Korean medicine through the establishment and operation of modern hospitals and the training of medical doctors.

The Joseon society and the government doubted the intentions of the early pioneering Western doctors and tried to suppress their activities. On the contrary, the Japanese rulers, during the Japanese colonial period, showed an amicable attitude. College education in medicine was therefore conducted systematically in this period and the graduation ceremony of the first 7 graduates of Severance Union Medical College (Currently, College of Medicine, Yonsei University) were the first medical license to practice Western medicine in Korea. This event shows that Western medicine was not rejected or expelled but continued to be accepted into the orthodox medicine during the Japanese colonial period.

2. Medical organization and market-oriented medical system in the Japanese colonial era

In particular, with the start of the Japanese colonial period, orthodox medicine was differentiated as clinics were categorized under the Decree on Clinics and differently classified from Western medicine. As a result, system of medicine in Korea was reorganized into a completely new form of medicine. Consequently, healthcare services were also reorganized, and the area emerged as a leading sector in acquiring modern features earlier than any other social and economic system in the Joseon Dynasty. Indeed, the starting point of Joseon medicine was based on foreign resources (human resources, facilities, equipment, and knowledge) and the paradigm introduced from the West. Accordingly, resources of the administrative school and the Daehan Medical Center during the late Joseon Dynasty, and Jahye Clinics under the Japanese Government－General of Korea were mobilized and distributed based on the decisions of the Japanese Government－General of Korea during the Japanese colonial era.

Thus, the policy characteristic was that it was already a system of national governance, and the most important public sectors were governed by the colonial government in Korea, together with the Japanese Government. In fact, the competitive establishment of hospitals by private−sector and public sector, especially the private sector, centered on Protestantism, which sought to penetrate Joseon society for gospel mission purposes, showed virtuous cycles in many aspects.

Following the Russian Revolution of 1917, the Soviet Semashko system (which was designed by Lenin's best friend Dr. Semashko to provide public healthcare to its people based on the most scientifically structured method), was adopted in some developing countries and other developed countries. However, the Korean healthcare system adopted a method that was run and supplied by market, except for the most essential necessities for survival, instead of a state−led system that dictated the operation of public healthcare related to medical doctors and medical care. The operation method of such system continued to expand supply and increased efficiency through competition between the private and public sectors, but the market function that the supply could accommodate the demand and need for healthcare service was preconditioned for growth.

3. Unmet needs for healthcare service

People in early days of modern Korea suffered from poverty and a number of infectious diseases. Waterborne infections, typhoid fever, tuberculosis, and leprosy were common diseases, and spread the of smallpox and Japanese encephalitis was rampant. Although the government provided basic supplies necessary for medical treatment, the medical services that could be provided to the public with the natural allocation of resources related to the actual operation of hospitals were extremely limited. Under the society of polarized distribution of wealth and privileges, the healthcare service was operated with the cycle of "the rich−get−richer and the poor−get−poorer" based on the market−oriented system, which was not beneficial to the overall public health. Therefore, in the Japanese colonial era, the agenda of popularizing doctors as a group of social leaders or elites during the doctor training process had been a subject of constant policy debate. In the curriculum for medical colleges and its process, controversy continued over how far the government should take the burden of the private sector and determine the level of doctors. However, elite doctors continued to be nurtured based on a social consensus that assuring the quality of doctors was critical and they should have considerable standard of medical knowledge and expertise upon graduation. The graduate doctors absorbed the society's constant demand for doctors and practiced medicine. The healthcare system also functioned as an important means of increasing their economic income level and accumulating assets.

4. Elevating the status of doctors and providing private-sector centered medical services

The substantial profits from the doctors' practice of medicine affected society through economic inflation. They then further increased their financial assets through investment activities, making themselves the next generation of the upper class of society. They would have been accustomed to their asset growth through continuous investment and expanded healthcare service. Operations in the public sector continued in the form of allocating certain proportion of national budgets, and the public sector grew to reflect the demands. Although the resources invested in the initial establishment and operation of public sector reflected the level of advanced system of developed countries, there was no significant increase in the operational efficiency or resource allocation. Therefore, the operation of public sector was based on maintaining the status quo or gradual decrease of the investment after reaching a certain level. The public and private healthcare share was 50-50 at the end of Japanese colonial era, especially because economic difficulties and war conditions reduced the state finances for allocating resources for healthcare service. Of course, in terms of resource allocation for medical schools, the public sector accounted for much more significant proportion than that of the private sector; butthe doctors, who graduated from the private or public universities and acquired medical license and underwent specialist training, were first hired in public institutions and then moved to private institutions after some time, thereby contributing to the promotion and development of private institutions. Increasingly, private sector−dominant markets were formed due to the expansion of the economic power of the doctors' group and their ability to mobilize assets, and the limited impact of the public sector's investment in healthcare. So, the healthcare market centered on private healthcare rather than public and this became a trend regardless of policy intentions. The training of doctors of oriental medicine, dentists, nurses, and medical technicians who were professional medical personnel in the healthcare sectors of Joseon was not active at the time, and it was not until after Korea's liberation from Japan that training for these professionals was properly implemented. In the field of healthcare, training of professionals, except for nurses, was carried out through an unregularized method of training necessary human resources at each hospital. The establishment of regular system was delayed until after Korea's liberation from Japan. In relation to healthcare facilities, hospitals were mainly established in the public sector rather than in the private sector, and the healthcare facilities in the private sector were not subject to legal orders. Therefore, private sector hospitals were poorly regulated and barely managed to treat or care for patients in empty spaces; subsequently, the infrastructure and facilities were built with an increase in their assets based on increased revenue. Reforms were carried out by establishing manpower and facilities necessary for practicing healthcare that could be prioritized over introduction of other specialized equipment. At that time, because supply for pharmaceuticals in the market was problematic, pharmaceutical industry or medical equipment industry did not show much growth. However, medicines that were essential for treatment of acute infectious diseases or for surgical procedures started to be imported. In the early days, drugs were imported mainly from Japan and Germany. It was also true that Japanese pharmaceutical companies entered Korea for drug manufacturing, imported pharmaceutical products from North American and European pharmaceutical companies, and laid the foundation for domestic production. To meet social demands, these drugs and medical supplies were produced and supplied at the appropriate level of Korean society rather than directly importing advanced products from the overseas. Centered around universities and associations of doctors and nurses, the efforts to improve the production and distribution of knowledge were known to social and medical fields, and these were formed through associations such as the Joseon association of doctors. Therefore, with medical schools at the center, the production and distribution of knowledge emerged as important issues. In this regard, the adoption of private sector system is an important reason for making public medical schools competitive.

Section 2
From 1945 to 1960s; Birth of Healthcare Policy

The modern healthcare system policy in Korea can be dated back to the 1945s. The healthcare sector became the most important part of society as the US military administration began during that period. After the establishment of the Korean government, the relevant government organization was launched on November 4, 1948, as the Ministry of Social Affairs, one of the 11 administrative agencies under the Government Organization Act. In February 1955, the Ministry of Health and the Ministry of Social Affairs were merged to form the Ministry of Health and Social Affairs. In addition, laws such as the National Medicine Services Law in 1951, the Law on Prevention of Communicable Diseases in 1954, the Law of Health Center establishment and operation in 1956, the Law on the prevention of Parasitic Diseases in 1966, and the Tuberculosis Prevention Act in 1968, were enacted and legal grounds were laid. At that time, the Jahye Clinics and the National University Hospital operated by the Japanese government were transferred to the Korean government. Thus, public sector healthcare was established, but existing private − sector healthcare was far short of meeting healthcare needs under the liberation regime. The private sector continued to expand the healthcare sector through the hospitals with supply systems and human resources practicing medicine as doctors. At this time, doctors and scholars in each field of expertise began to launch academic research organizational societies to develop their fields. As a result, the foundation on which knowledge resources in medical education and research could spread to have an impact on society started to be established after 1885.

The Korean War from 1950 to 1953 destroyed most public and private medical facilities and interrupted healthcare services. Efforts to rebuild and standardize healthcare at an appropriate level were still challenging. Even though it was during the Korean War, efforts to constantly promote research on medicine and improve the level of practice in medicine could be made, thanks to foreign support. To train health professional for public health, various organizations, including the World Health Organization (WHO), the China Medical Board (CMB), the Population Council, and the Korea − U.S. Foundation, provided financial support and aid. Many health professionals applied to pursue master's degrees in healthcare studies, mainly in the U.S.

The National Medical Center was established in 1958 to restore ruins across the country with medical staff and medical equipment support from the Scandinavian countries. As a result, medical staff from Northern Europe were dispatched to Korea, and some medical staff from South Korea were also trained in Northern Europe. Through the private sector missionary network, Korean doctors learned advanced medicine in the U.S. and some continued their medical careers in the U.S. Medical school education in Korea and the U.S. were set to a similar level because Medical doctor from Korea had to meet the required medical school graduation standards in order to become a doctor in the U.S. Also, the Korea National Tuberculosis Association in 1953 and the Korean Leprosy Association in 1956 were established that linked private and public sectors in the fight against theses diseases. The dental college for regular dental training was first established in 1959 by the Department of Dentistry of Seoul National University, and 8 years later, dental colleges were established at Yonsei University and Kyung Hee University. The oriental medical school, which was removed after the Japanese colonial era, was established in 1964 in Dongyang University as a six−year program of oriental medicine, and Kyung Hee University's oriental medical major, established in 1965, was developed into an oriental medical school in 1976. In addition, the nursing training course began at the Boguyeogwan in Jeong−dong, and after Korea's liberation from Japanese colonial rule, the department of nursing welfare within the Haenglimwon was formed in 1947 and the department of nursing education was established in 1950. In 1955, the first undergraduate program of nursing department in Korea was approved at Yonsei and Ewha Womans Universities, and the graduate school opened a master's degree program in the 1960s. At that time, it was practically difficult for people to visit hospitals and clinics for medical treatment because they had difficulty paying for medical expenses. Therefore, it was quite challenging for the government to invest funds in the public sector to install medical facilities and supply medical equipment and supplies. The government's active efforts in the healthcare sector were made through a five−year economic development plan in 1962 and carried out in a way that could revitalize the healthcare market and meet demand. In 1960, Korea had a birth rate of 6.0, and since 1961, a strong family planning project was carried out by the government to to control population growth[1] for economic development.

At that time, it was difficult to revitalize the market without government investment, but the family planning project was carried out in hopes of increasing gross product by reducing the population. The family planning project, which began as a social movement, was funded by the International Planned Parenthood Federation (IPPF) along with the government budget of the health and medical sectors, and was carried out through the private sector's Family Planning Association. The family planning projects were funded by various foreign institutions, which contributed to the expansion of the medical market by people who were consumers and healthcare workers who were providers. In 1963, the government contributed to the private sector, including medical practices such as intrauterine devices (IUD), a method of contraception for women, by allocating funds for family planning projects. In addition, family planning projects contributed greatly to the expansion of the public sector's

---

1) Jang, et al. (2010), Korea's Population Policy: History and Future, Korea Institute for Health and Social Affairs.

organization and workforce.

Since 1950, health centers had many difficulties in carrying out healthcare projects due to the lack of medical professionals. In particular, in rural areas, where it was difficult to hire medical doctors for medical institutions, institutional policies were set for placement of health workers and public service doctors, to perform family planning services, mother and child health healthcare, and tuberculosis management. In the 1960s, Korean society was in the state of absolute poverty, so economic growth was the main priority. As a result, policy interest in the health and welfare sector was weak, but this period can be said to be a time when the legislative system was established and institutionalized.

Section 3
From 1970s to 1980s; Expanding Healthcare Policies

1. Overview

The history of healthcare policy shifted from the era of family planning to the era of health insurance. Economic development was achieved at a remarkable pace from a per capita gross national income (GNI) of $80 in 1960, to $257 in 1970, and to $1,686 in 1980. In 1977, the year when the national income was $1,000 per person, the health insurance system was started and the Korean population started to apply since 1989. The 1970s and 1980s, the period when the government actively promoted expansion of public welfare, were period of great significance in the healthcare sectors. At that time, 42 million policyholders for national health insurance represented the entire population except for 3 million including soldiers. Previous family planning projects had significant impact on medical demand or healthcare providers, allowing the healthcare system to develop and move forward. Overseas funds allowed experimental facilities for universities and research to be set up, and especially with the cooperation of Japan, popularization of medical supplies began.

2. Influence of the Family planning projects

The newly established Family Planning Office and Maternity and Child Welfare Office under the Ministry of Health and Welfare (MOHW) were promoted to Maternity and Child Welfare Management Office in 1972. The Office was able to establish three divisions, Family Planning Division, Maternity and Child Welfare Division, and National Nutrition Division, and implemented basic international businesses. The works of police, sanitary management and administration were transferred or separated. The health and medical service network, which did not meet the public healthcare needs for a long time, expanded to farming and fishing villages. The government contributed to family planning projects that were appropriate for economic conditions at that time and that could derive aid and loan from foreign countries instead of implementing health insurance, which was impracticable to be expanded. The family planning project contributed to two levels: first, establishing a public organization that can provide basic healthcare services, and second, growing a new medical market based on revitalized private healthcare. Instead of providing medical services directly for the public health service, private medical institutions were encouraged to participate. It boosted the private market, which had been suffering from lack of demand, while increasing the effectiveness of the private medical business and reducing costs. The new workforce, which was supplied to the market to grow and became an important policy subject. And one of the policy objectives, permanent contraception, was considered the most effective policy direction, and fiscal spending was effectively achieved when permanent contraception was done. This boosted the healthcare market by expanding the public sector and the private market. Previously, it was difficult for the public to access medical care, but the popularization of medical care began by improving public access to medical care through the government's family planning projects. The awareness of medical care, which was relatively unfamiliar, was improved so that people could use it comfortably. That is, the family planning project eased the public burden of using hospitals and reduced obstacles to the use of medical services by the general public. The military also created medical demand. At that time, the public healthcare organizations were expanded to establish local health center networks and increased the supply of health professionals in all areas, including disease control. The public sector minimized what had to be provided by doctors and the private sector participated in the provision of medical services.

3. Introduction and management of the National Health Insurance System

Based on the above, health insurance was finally ready for implementation. The key starting point of the transition of health insurance from the era of family planning was that facilities and equipment were developed and financed by Japan. If this amount of money had been used as health insurance in the first place instead of healthcare industry, the money would not have been able to be invested in the healthcare industry. In 1962, national health insurance began to be introduced at a level of $1,000 gross national income per capita (PPP), as the income of the people increased, thanks to the medical industry used for public welfare[2]. The biggest impact of family planning was the increased demand for healthcare service. In the first five-year family planning healthcare, the investment was focused on improving doctorless villages, increasing medical equipment, building new local health centers and improving city and provincial hospitals, but the policy establishment and investment on expansion of medical facilities were lacking. In addition, as investment in medical facilities properly began in the 5th and 6th Economic and Social Development Planning era (1982-1991), experimental equipment was installed in some universities and hospitals through foreign borrowing or loan. Since the use of the facility in private facilities could turn into a money-making project, the priority in allocation of foreign loan was selected for university research experiment and testing facilities, and the facilities that were rarely available in local community. In this way, Japan's advanced level of medical devices were introduced to Korea based on overseas funds, and the

---

2) Kim Young-Suk et al. (2007), Health insurance and economic growth, Health insurance forum 2007 Winter.

domestic medical service sector was expanded as the existing domestic medical services alone could not handle the situation. As a result, great medical advances were made as the time was reduced with the help of automated devices, while people once had to wait for a long time because previously blood tests were run one by one. In addition, medical devices that could conduct radiation tests, blood tests, and microbiological tests were introduced through overseasborrowing. Among medical devices imported from abroad, Japanese products were more competitive than other countries' and had a structure suitable for the situation in Korea, contributing greatly to the development of domestic medical equipment and medical products. Although high–end medical devices such as U.S. products were also imported, Japanese medical devices were used commonly, and they were practically suitable for Korean medical environment. This led to diversification and popularization of healthcare services. However, it was in the very early stages to diversity medical services, due to the old facilities, such as medical facilities and medical equipment that exixted and the thelack of doctors. Also, there were no facilities to manufacture drugs. For this reason, the private market created a system of demand and more people wanted to trade in the system. In 1963, the medical insurance took a very basic form and was used in the public sector mainly by dispatching doctors to local health centers. This is because it was operated in a way to subsidize the private sector. In 1977, various healthcare services were provided by the private sector, and operating rates, in which the private sector was competitive against the public sector, were boosted by new technologies introduced at the time. The public satisfaction increased by receiving the service from the private sector. Therefore, this was why the public was highly receptive when health insurance services were introduced.

At the proposal of the Social Security Discussion Committee within the Ministry of Health and Social Affairs in February 1963, the draft Medical Insurance Act was to apply health insurance to workplaces with more than 500 employees. Therefore, in December 1976, the Medical Insurance Act was fully revised, which called for the application of health insurance by default. Based on this, the nation's health insurance system was first implemented in July 1977 for workers at workplaces with more than 500 employees. Afterwards, the government felt the financial burden of health insurance and changed the application to the voluntary application of workplaces with more than 300 employees. At that time, economic and social requirements were poor, and the medical market was difficult to revitalize without investment. In addition, self–employed people had a huge problem with health insurance. Therefore, the occupational union membership was formed. Korea's population was a structural system in which high–income earners and low–income earners existed. In 1977, the government established a foundation for health insurance by implementing a medical insurance system in the form of state responsibility for 10% of low–income families. At that time, the medical system was allocated a considerable amount of funds of 9.6 billion won. Although the fee of the medical insurance was set to be lower than the general charges, it was a system that was welcomed by rural medical institutions and low–income medical service consumers because the system offered free medical services to low–income populations. In the case of North Korea at that time, the health insurance system was already introduced and provided free medical care. As a result, South Korea had no choice but to create and introduce a social security system for medical service in some form amid a very strong inter–Korean competitive situation. Medical insurance was provided to all people except for 10% of medical aid beneficiaries in 1989, after 12 years of its introduction in 1977. So, as the national income level rose and healthcare service providers were stabilized, service capabilities improved for enhanced satisfaction of the public. As a result, since people could contribute to medical expenses on their own, more people used hospitals through health insurance benefits, and access to hospitals increased. Thus, the current health insurance plan could be achieved. The medical charge could be lower than the standard compared to medical costs, but the income was increased due to rising demand for actual use of medical service. The 1977 medical insurance scheme was a remarkable one, as providers were able to accept the financial aspect of the medical insurance policy. As a result, the possibility of expanding the medical insurance coverage to medical service with high excellence began to gradually decrease. Although the quality of medical care provided by the insurance coverage alone was reduced, the quality was to be maintained in consideration of the public interests. Therefore, the coverage rate rose as the service covered by medical insurance increased from 40 to 50 percent at first to 55 percent, 60 percent, and to 70 percent. These are the key reasons for the growth of Korean medical service.

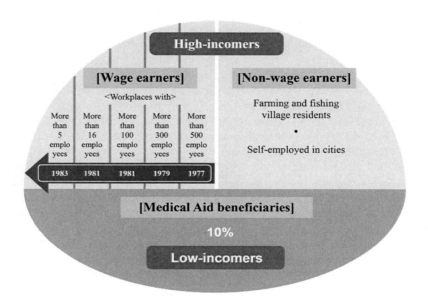

〈Figure 1〉 Health Care System from Medical Insurance Act

In September 1976, the 'plan to expand medical benefits to improve public health' was officially announced, and a plan to institutionalize medical benefits for low−income families and the foundation for national healthcare were established. Thus, the Medical Care Act was enacted in December 1977 and established an institutional framework for two major pillars of medical insurance and medical care.

The nation's medical insurance system underwent a number of changes until the 'National Health Insurance (NHI)' was introduced in July 1989. With the start of urban regional health insurance on 1 July 1989, the 'National Health Insurance (NHI)' was formally implemented. The coverage of the health insurance for the entire Korean population continued to increase and the debate over how to manage today's healthcare system continued.

With the establishment of the health insurance system, the medical service market began to grow as it expanded not only to existing supply systems but also to those who provided new supplies. These medical service consumers wanted diversification in participants of medical service providers. At that time, only medical personnel could establish hospitals or clinics, but health insurance enabled providers other than medical personnel to establish hospitals in rural areas. Therefore, non−profit corporations, such as medical corporations, were qualified to establish hospitals. In 1983-84, the establishment of hospitals by medical personnel has competitive strength, but the establishment of private hospitals as non−profit corporations by non−medical personnel was not managed by the principle of market. Hospitals were linked to medical schools and had limitations in paying by private investment in establishing hospitals. Therefore, the government arranged foreign loans with low interest rates. The loans could only be used for corporations of public good, and policies were created that purchases were limited to equipment and essential supplies and luxury goods were not allowed to be purchased. Therefore, investment was concentrated on the healthcare sector and growth began. The question of costs for medical demand was a question of whether it would be possible to earn proper profits by tailoring suppliers according to effective demand methods and prevent large profits for individual operators. There was no problem with the operation of small hospitals and small profits as individual businesses, but people who run large hospitals were required to verify their accounting plans, as a public surveillance function. In these formats and methods, the support and development of private medical institutions were increased and strengthened.

4. Overcoming contradictions in the healthcare system

The issue of equity in medical service supply was extremely important in Korea. In order to resolve the problem of inequality in medical service provision in vulnerable areas, the 'Doctorless village policy' began with collected opinions that "there should be at least one doctor" in each city and county's vulnerable areas. In 1961 military coup, the Republican military forced those who did not join the military to serve in a doctorless village, and those who wanted to immigrate abroad had to serve as the head of a local health center for a year. In addition, in order to address the doctorless village issue, residents were required to work in a doctorless village for six months during a four−year training period to qualify for a specialist exam. That is, in December 1971, the government took the issue of medical service supply shortage in doctorless villages, and in 1972, a dispatching medical resident system started operation. Residents had to mandatorily work in doctorless village for six months out of four years of their major courses to qualify for a specialist exam. They were required to work in farming and fishing villages for six months and ordered to work in a doctorless village. Later, the government began to deploy public health doctors to doctorless villages from 1981 to address the problem of supply in medical service. In December 1983, with Docheon－myeon, Changnyeong－gun, Gyeongsangnam－do as the last, a total of 1,503 public health doctors were assigned to doctorless villages and the problem of doctorless village was completely resolved.

Section 4

From 1990s to 2000s; Ongoing Efforts to Improve the Quality of Life for the Public

1. Attempts to meet the demand for medical service through cultivation of health professionals

In order to understand the history of development of Korean healthcare system, it is first necessary to consider the fact that modern Korea started out as one of the least developed countries and therefore, investment of resources in healthcare sector had been neglected from priorities. As part of attempts to meet demand for healthcare services with minimal financial input, the government granted permission for foundation of medical schools. In 1990, the government revised the process of granting permission for medical schools, but the number of the schools had already increased rapidly between 1970s – 1980s. The main reason was the demand for health professionals in doctorless villages. Therefore, with the establishment of new medical schools continued in the late 1970s, and in the early 1980s, the number of medical schools sharply increased, resulting in the production of a large number of medical personnel. At that time, the establishment of a university underwent the approval process, but from 1990 in the government of President Kim Young – Sam, a normative system was introduced on university establishment under which the university establishment was granted by reporting whether the new university to be established satisfies the minimum requirements on facilities and manpower. This regulation reform led to the establishment of a myriad of universities simply because the founder wanted the status of chief director of a university. Following this change in university establishment in 1970s – 1990s, there were around 3,200 new graduates every year from 42 medical colleges. Still, there were medical doctors who accumulated their wealth to the level of capitalists. However, nowadays, as the values of doctors have changed in various aspects, there are now more doctors conducting research or teaching in medical colleges and fewer who accumulate wealth to become capitalists. As a result, a layperson is entitled to establish medical schools and hospitals instead of medical doctors.

2. Separation of dispensary from medical practice and financial crisis in national health insurance budget

Separation of dispensary from medical practice, whose principle originated from the enactment of the Pharmaceutical Affairs Act in 1953, was implemented after half a century. On July 1, 2000, in the year of the new millennium, separation of dispensary from medical practice was first implemented in Korea. Due to the implementation of the separation, which is regarded one of the representative headline issues in the field of healthcare since 1990, there was a total chaotic crisis in health insurance finances, leading to a deficit in the balance. Despite decades of discussion and forming of social consensus in the process of implementation between the government and interest groups, the barrier due to differences between the interest groups seemed almost insurmountable. Although the process of reconciling the differences with the government, medical doctors and pharmacists faced several obstacles such as extreme oppositions from both doctors and pharmacists, separation of dispensary from medical practice was implemented in full backed up by strong determination of the government in July 1999. As a result, doctors went on a strike in protest, completely shutting down their practice for the first week of implementing the separation policy. The protest continued later even after they withdrew their initial protest and there was another strike which caused a complete chaos in medical service. In order to resolve this ongoing conflict, since September 6, 2000, the government had discussion meetings with doctors 26 times and 8 times with pharmacists. As a result, on October 31, 2000, the government reached a comprehensive agreement on the additional complementary measures for implementation of the separation of dispensary from medical practice in November 2000, through Korean Medical Association and Korean Pharmaceutical Association[3]. Since then, the system of separation of dispensary from medical practice entered the phase of stabilization in implementation.

Immediately after the implementation, the finances of the national health insurance were faced with great difficulties. This was because the 139 workplace insurance unions, which started in November 2000, were completely integrated with the National Health Insurance Service, and through the implementation of separation of dispensary from medical practice, insurance benefit cost increased sharply compared to revenue from health insurance contributions. For this reason, the finances of national health insurance resulted in a deficit in the year 2001 with a surge in insurance benefit costs. The deficit amounted to KRW 2.5 trillion in 2001 but turned to a surplus of KRW 1 trillion in 2003.

Accordingly, Ministry of Health and Welfare (MOHW) proposed various countermeasures through 'Financial Prospects of National Health Insurance and Measures for Stable Operation of Finances' for stabilized running of the finances of health insurance. In January 2002, a national health promotion charge was imposed on cigarettes, and for raising national health promotion fund, Special Act on Sound Finance of National Health

---

3) MOHW, Proposal on Amendment of Pharmaceutical Affairs Act through Agreement between Medical Sector, Pharmaceutical Sector, and Government. (2000.12.11. Press Release)
    http://www.mohw.go.kr/react/al/sal0301vw.jsp?PAR_MENU_ID=04&MENU_ID=0403&page=983&CONT_SEQ=19557

Insurance was enacted in which the management operational fee and insurance benefit cost of locally provided policyholders are supported from the national treasury fund.

3. Establishment of a healthcare system in response to changes in the social and demographic structure

After historical changes as described above, health insurance coverage was further expanded by implementing the long–term care insurance system for the elderly with diseases such as dementia and stroke. Efforts to enhance health insurance coverage include reducing co–payments for patients with severe illness, and those with rare and intractable diseases, improving health insurance coverage rate through the application of denture insurance for the elderly, expanding coverage for four major diseases, and improving the national health checkup system to strengthen the proactive preventive management system and significantly strengthening the safety management system to prepare for new diseases and emergencies.

In addition, in 2011, continuous efforts for development of the healthcare industry were made such as enactment of Special Act on Fostering and Support of Pharmaceutical Industry, strategic expansion of national R&D to foster the medical device industry, and establishment of Daegu–Gyeongbuk Medical Innovation Foundation for enhancement of quality of life for the national population. However, Korea still falls short of the level of developed countries, and there are remaining challenges for Korean healthcare industry such as measures to reduce medical expenses that increase the level of health insurance coverage, establishment of health care delivery system, and resolving imbalances in medical services between regions.

Period	Health product industry	Healthcare industry
Short-term (2000-2002)	Building a foundation for self-reliance	Establishment of an institutional base
Middle-term (2003-2005)	Establishing a foundation for self-reliance	Fiscal consolidtion and equity enhancement
Long-term (2006-2010)	Leap forward as a self-reliant country	Provision of quality medical services
Final	Industrial independence	Advancement of Healthcare industry
	Strengthening international competitiveness and improving the quality of life of the people through development as a core strategic project of knowledge-based economic society in the 21st century	

〈Figure 2〉 Development objectives of Korea's health industry in stages

※ Source: DA1046561, p.11

The medical fee system in the 1970s focused on lowered fee than the actual rate to improve public access, and from the 1990s to the 2000s, the fee–for–service system was in operation. After the decision to introduce relative value medical fee in 1994, medical service demand surged in 2000 according to the policy to expand health insurance coverage through normalization of medical fee through relative value. In addition to the implementation of separation of dispensary from medical practice, the financial balance of national health insurance turned into a deficit due to the significant cost of medical service. Therefore, countermeasures were taken at the policy level to address the problem of deficit. In addition, with the implementation of long−term care insurance, the medical expenditure of Korea rose from 5−6% of gross domestic product (GDP) to 7.6% in 2018, which is still lower than the OECD average of 8.8%, but is increasing at a rapid pace[4]. In fact, in terms of covered medical expenditure and non−covered medical expenditure, the coverage level of Korea has been maintained at the highest level among countries of similar economic status. In 2018, the ratio of annual outpatient treatment per capita was 16.9%, the highest among OECD countries. That is, the rate of use of hospital service is 2.5 times higher than the OECD average of 6.8%[5].

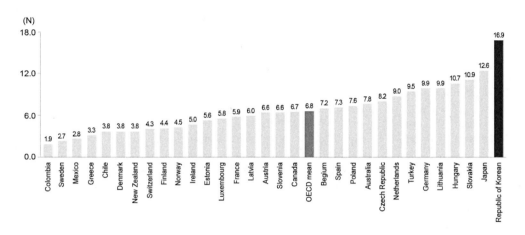

⟨Figure 3⟩ Number of outpatients visits per capita (2018)

※ Source: MOHW (2019), OECD Health Statistics 2020, MOHW press release

In the past, continuous efforts have been made to expand health insurance coverage, increase coverage of chronic diseases, and provide more medical facilities, but until the late 1990s, the number of beds in medical institutions was small. Previously, because medical technology was offered at a low price, the health insurance fee increased the amount of claims, and in order to increase the amount collected from patients' contribution, a large number of services as seen in the list of medical service such as imaging equipment, clinical diagnostic equipment, and laboratory diagnostic equipment were delivered to the public. The reason is that numerous medical devices were imported through foreign aid or loan, and medical services that were thought to

---

4) Song, Seok−Eun (2020), A study on competition and antitrust issues in the pharmaceutical sector, Law School, Sungkyunkwan University, Ph.D. thesis.

5) MOHW (2019), OECD Health Statistics 2020, MOHW press release.

be effective for application through the use of medical devices were included in the medical services, and thus the medical fee increased the overall cost of treatment. Now, through health insurance coverage, the public access to medical service has increased. For the general public, the price barrier for medical care is not high and actually, the country now has the highest accessibility to medical service compared to other countries. Doctors can earn income through patients who use medical services, and since the number of patients is large compared to the per capita productivity of doctors in other countries, doctors in Korea can treat a greater number of patients. This has led to an increase in the number of outpatient and inpatient services. In the past, as the quality of care continued to increase, there was a tendency to set the scope and quantity of treatment care much more and higher than necessary. At first, strong policy measures to suppress such tendency were used, but it was difficult to implement such a policy due to the alliance between the supplier and the consumer. In addition, with a large increase in the demand for welfare, the long−term care insurance, which was not previously included in the medical insurance in the past and the current health insurance, has still not been resolved, but since the welfare for the nursing care for the elderly falls under the long−term care insurance, it is still part of the area of public health. If the coverage can go beyond the long−term care insurance and cover the nursing care for the elderly, this would correspond to welfare and the system will be expanded to the public health welfare system.

As for the background of implementing long−term care insurance, the demographic structure has changed sharply, and we have entered the era of population aging with a large number of elderly people. Japan prepared for the era of nursing care facilities for the elderly early through the Gold plan[6] for the elderly in 1989. Through comparison and a review of Japanese policies in many areas of healthcare policy, Korea will develop policy with more dramatic effects. In the overall consideration of healthcare system, with more elderly retiring from their work, the demand for hospitalization and nursing care facilities increased. Unlike acute diseases, the demand for chronic diseases will increase in terms of chronic diseases management, and beds for long−term care of chronic diseases, which are different from those for acute diseases, will be needed. In establishing a long−term care hospital, it is necessary to consider at what level the long−term care insurance should be set and the scope of public investment. The most important point is the government developing a plan for financing and utilization of the finances and not constructing facilities for long−term care for public investment. In addition, it should be possible to build nursing care facilities in areas with limited development such as green belts across the country.

Nursing hospitals and nursing homes will be supported by the method of public sector and financing will be provided in a number of areas to run the service, and thus, a large number of beds will be supplied from the public sector. As a result, the number of beds for nursing hospitals and nursing homes will increase significantly through long−term care insurance, and in this case, Korea will have the largest number of beds in relation to the population size when compared with other countries worldwide.

---

6) Choi, E.K. et al. (2005), Issues in long−term care services in OECD countries and policy implications for Korea, Korea Institute for Health and Social Affairs.

When examining the clinical setting of Korea due to COVID−19 pandemic this time, hospitals and beds in Korea were constructed and made with reference to foreign standards but the standards for healthcare facilities of Korea have not been revised. This is because, when the standards for healthcare facilities are revised, the expansion is not possible when the set standards are not satisfied, so the priority has been on the expansion of facilities by accepting resources from public sector rather than setting the standards and quality of excellence. To this end, the required investment for facilities should be reduced while maximizing the effect of supply. Since the government does not make any profit, it was initially implemented through the method of attracting capitals from public sector, especially medical personnel. However, since medical personnel do not tend to make much investment due to their nature, healthcare facilities should be established as non−for−profit corporation and the investment from public sector should be drawn while ensuring their profitability. In this process, the hospitals were not required to provide good level of facilities and the standards for healthcare facilities were not properly established. Therefore, even the standards for medical personnel such as number of patients served per doctor and nurse, and other personnel required for running of health facilities were not strictly determined. Only recently, the supply has been sufficiently ensured and it was possible to raise the standards of healthcare facilities to increase the standard of health insurance benefits and therefore, the standards for hospital facilities and medical personnel have been revised. In this way, the current standards for hospital facilities and medical personnel were developed.

4. Awareness on Industrialization of Healthcare Service

In the 1990s and 2000s, the Ministry of Health and Welfare (MOHW) developed various types of projects to foster the health industry as a strategic project for the 21st century. The 'Health and Medical Technology Research and Development Project' started since February 1995, and the results of joint research conducted by the Korea Institute for Health and Social Affairs and the Korea Health Industry Development Institute for around 6 months from May to October were reported to MOHW. In December of the same year, the Health and Medical Service Technology Promotion Act was enacted with the purpose of contributing to the sound development of the healthcare industry and the promotion of public health.

In January 1997, the 'mid−and long−term development plan for health and medical technology' was established and active efforts were made for R&D projects worth 1.5 trillion won. "A Study on Establishment of 21st Century Health Industry Development Strategy" was jointly conducted by Korea Health Industry Development Institute and Korea Institute for Health and Social Affairs, which focused on the following areas: future prospects of the social and economic environment of the health industry (prospects for supply and demand in the health industry, outlook on the health industry environment); the importance and status of the health industry; the current status and problems of the health industry in Korea; comparison and analysis of Korea and Japan health industry; strategic evaluation of health industry in Korea; current status and implications of domestic and overseas health industry promotion policies; health industry development strategies; health industry development strategy promotion system; and vision and comprehensive structural design of the 21st century

Korean health industry (Yeom, Yong—Gwon, 1999)[7]. Accordingly, the Korea Health Industry Development Institute was established in 1999 for professional and systematic support of projects for the promotion and development of the Korean health industry and the improvement of healthcare services based on the enactment of the Korea Health Industry Development Institute Act.

Also, in November 1994, the Osong Health and Medical Science Complex was established to foster the healthcare industry as the 21st century national core strategic project based on the 'Innovation Plan for Health and Medical Science and Technology' of MOHW. In line with the plan, starting from the groundbreaking ceremony in October 2003, the Osong Bio—Health Science Technopolis was completed in October 2008. Since then, as of 2020, the six National Policy Institutes [(Korea Disease Control and Prevention Agency (KDCA), National Institute of Food and Drug Safety Evaluation (NFDS), Korea National Institute of Health, Ministry of Food and Drug Safety (MFDS), Korea Health Industry Development Institute, Korea Human Resource Development Institute for Health & Welfare)] and 61 private corporations signed the lease agreements for occupancy, and the place has established itself as the hub of healthcare industry in Korea.

---

7) Yeom, Yong—Gwon (1999), A Study on Establishment of 21st Century Health Industry Development Strategy.

Chapter 2

Changes in policies for providing medical services in Korea

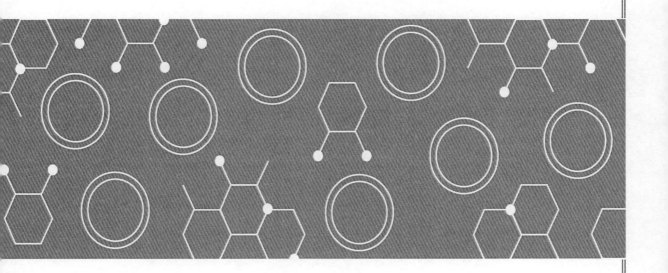

Section 1

Establishment of Public Health System

1. Public Health System

The United States Army Military Government in Korea (USAMGIK), which set out in South Korea after the liberation on August 15, promulgated the "Bill on the Establishment of a Sanitation Bureau" as USAMGIK Ordinance No. 1 on September 24, 1945, in an attempt to establish an independent Sanitary Bureau[8] promoting preventive public health projects.

The public health projects kick−started in October, 1946, with the establishment of a model public health center in Seoul, which was promoted to the National Health Center after the establishment of the Republic of Korea. With aid from the United Nations, 15 public health centers and 471 community health posts were established in 1953[9], playing a pivotal role in regional health administration. In December 1956, Korea enacted and promulgated the "Public Health Center Act[10]", and established and operated public health centers and health subcenters in about 500 places across the country, formalizing the public health center business. However, the health centers were properly organized due to shortage of budget. In September 1962, the "Public Health Center Act" was completely amended, and public health centers were deployed in provinces and cities across the country, forming a systematic health and medical network[11]. In 1969, 1,336 health subcenters were installed in rural areas (eup or myeon), but there were difficulties in securing a health care workforce and facility equipment[12].

---

8) Yang Il−seok (2015), The Story of Veterinary Medicine in Modern Korean History(3), Journal of the Korean Veterinary Medical Association, p.465

9) Lee Dong−won (2020), The Korean War and the formation of Korean "Public Health", Dongguk Historical Society vol.69, p.355

10) Son Myung−se, The State and Medicine in Korea in the 20th Century: Health Care System, Journal of the Korean Medical Association, 제vol.42 no.12. p.1156

11) Korean Cultural History, Changes in Public Health Policies and Their Impact on Daily Life. http://contents.history.go.kr/front/km/print.do?levelId=km_004_0060_0040_0030_0020&whereStr=

12) Kang Bok−soo (2000), Improvement of Public Health Services in Korea, p.220

〈Table 1〉 Annual Trends of Public Health Centers and Community Health Posts

Year	Public Health Center	Primary Health Care Post
1953	15	471
1954	16	470
1955	16	515
1956	17	505
1957	22	513
1958	26	499
1959	68	–
1960	80	–
1961	87	–
1962	189	–

※ Source: Seoul Health Research Society, Health White Paper vol.1, 1981, p.21

General hospitals and city and provincial hospitals were operated until the end of 1960 to play a leading role in health care service policy. However, as time passed, the public health care sector fell far behind in terms of facilities, workforce, and other financial resources compared to the private health care sector. In the health care market led by private health care institutions, the imbalance in health care resources between regions deepened, and the government distributed public health care management tasks to eight ministries.

In January 1977, starting with the medical insurance project, the primary, secondary, and tertiary health care institutions were designated to establish a patient referral system. Primary health care institutions included public health centers, health subcenters, community health posts, and designated private practices treating outpatients. Secondary health care institutions include designated private hospitals as well as city and provincial hospitals treating outpatients. Tertiary health care institutions included national hospitals treating patients.

After the introduction of medical insurance in 1977, the nationwide medical insurance system was partially implemented in 1989, resulting in a sharp increase in health care demand[13]. Compared to private hospitals, public hospitals desperately needed investment in outdated facilities. For this, the "City and Provincial Hospital Operation Improvement Planning Group" was organized from May to December 1981 under the supervision of the Office for Government Policy Coordination. Afterwards, the measures to improve public health care services at public health centers, city and provincial hospitals, and national university hospitals were discussed through public hearings.

---

13) National Health Insurance Research Institute (2020), The Necessity and Strategy of Expanding Public Health Care, p.1

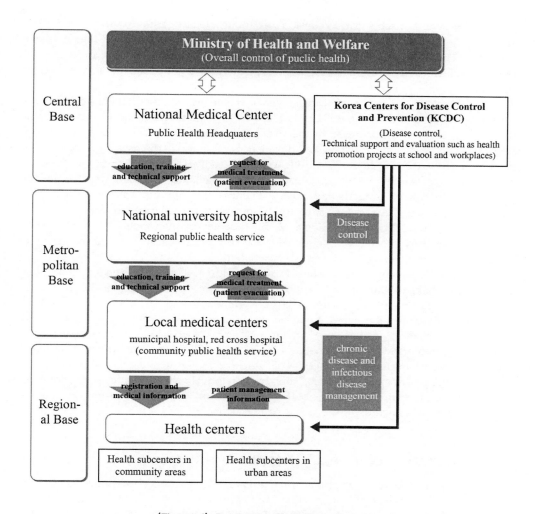

〈Figure 4〉 Public Health Delivery System

※ Source: Choo Ki-sook (2015), 70 years of Health and Welfare

In the 2000s, health care institutions in small and medium-sized cities and rural areas failed to contribute to an improvement in access to health care for the general public as the profitability of hospitals deteriorated, along with a shortage of health care workforce. Accordingly, in 2005, through pan-government discussions, the health care system was reformed as the "Comprehensive Measures for Expansion of Public Health," which served as an opportunity to expand public health care. Therefore, an investment in public health of KRW 4 trillion was decided over five years (2005 to 2009).

In June 2005, the "Act on the Establishment and Management of Local Medical Centers" was passed, and local medical centers were converted to the management and supervision system of the Ministry of Health and Welfare. Based on the

"Comprehensive Measures for Expansion of Public Health" announced in December 2005, the Red Cross Hospitals and local medical centers were fostered as regional base hospitals. The Red Cross Hospitals and local medical centers are now in charge of public health services through the medical safety net function for the medically vulnerable in the region[14].

The problems of the health care system revealed in the Comprehensive Measures for the Expansion of Public Health included, first, the inefficiency due to the failure of the market; second, the increase in the national health care burdens due to the aging population as well as the increased prevalence of chronic diseases; and third, the weak supply base of essential health care. To solve this problem, we secured modernized facility equipment, information technology, and excellent manpower for public hospitals, and strengthened competitiveness through innovation support and management analysis. Accordingly, the establishment of a public health delivery system with a central base hospital (National Medical Center) → metropolitan base hospitals (national university hospitals) → regional base hospitals (local medical centers) → communities (health centers, etc.) was carried out[15].

Through an amendment to the "Public Health and Medical Services Act," the government changed the focus of public health from "ownership" to "function." It stated, "all activities of the State, local governments, and of public and medical institutions to ensure all citizens equal access to medical services and to protect and promote their health, irrespective of which region they live in and to whatsoever class they belong," to include the activities of private health care institutions. Therefore, classifying the characteristics in terms of function rather than the establishment or operating entity can provide legal support for private health care institutions to perform public health care. The health care system is also premised on mutual complementation with the private health care sector.

2. Promotion of Primary Health Care Projects

It has been declared that primary health care (PHC) should be applied at various levels with the aim of the protection and promotion of global health and the resolution of inequality through the 1978 Alma−Ata Declaration (Cueto M, 2004)[16].

The government enacted the "Act on Special Measures for Public Health and Medical Services" in 1978 to address primary health problems in rural areas. The key content of this was to prepare a public health doctor system for the villages with no doctors. These measures included a plan to let those who passed the medical qualification examination among those waiting to join the military service, with no prior record of serving as a military doctor, serve as public health doctors at health subcenters in villages with no doctors in the 1960s. In addition, residents across the

---

14) Korea Health Industry Development Institute (2006), Measures to Strengthen the Publicity and Operational Efficiency of Regional Base Public Hospitals such as Regional Medical Centers, Policy−Health Care−2006−97.

15) Ministry of Welfare, "70 Years of Health and Welfare" vol.2 Health Care, 2016.

16) Cueto M. (2004), "The ORIGINS of Primary Health Care and SELECTIVE Primary Health Care". 《American Journal of Public Health》 94(11): 1864-1874. PMC 1448553.

country were given the qualifications to take the specialist exam only after serving in villages with no doctors for six months during their four years of training. The government began to deploy public health doctors in the villages with no doctors in 1981 to fundamentally solve the health care supply and demand problems in rural areas. In December 1983, a total of 1,503 public health doctors were dispatched to the villages with no doctors, ending with Docheon−myeon, Changnyeong−gun, Gyeongnam, thereby resolving the issues associated with the villages with no doctors. However, it was still difficult to meet all the health care needs in rural areas and enhance health care services in rural areas with the public health doctor system alone, and a new health care workforce was required.

With the enactment of the "Act on Special Measures for Health and Medical Services in Agricultural and Fishing Villages, Etc." in December 1980, the basis for intensively deploying public health doctors in vulnerable "agricultural and fishing village" areas among the villages with no doctors was laid (Jeong Gi−hye, 2017)[17]. The community health practitioner system has great significance for the primary health project in Korea, which has been continuously discussed since the 1960s in terms of implementing practical national health care policies in the local community to meet essential health care needs and expand public health services.

3. Establishment of Emergency Medical Service System

As Korea undergoes industrialization, emergency patients have started to occur constantly due to various accidents, such as industrial and traffic accidents, as well as diseases.

As a result of economic expansion, there was a social demand for an emergency medical system around 1980. Several deaths of emergency patients caused by the refusal of treatment in large hospitals have emerged as social problems. In July 1990, the implementation of national health insurance for the public led to an increase in the demand for health care from patients. Accordingly, the possibility of acute emergency disease or damage has increased due to various types of accidents and disasters, along with a surge in traffic volume, an increased prevalence of adult diseases, and an aging population In addition, as mass disasters have started to occur more frequently, the need to establish a disaster emergency medical system as well as a pre−hospital phase emergency medical system has increased.

In 1990, the Ministry of Health and Social Affairs held the "Committee on Emergency Medical System." As a result, 79 emergency medical centers were designated nationwide, with health care workers on standby 24 hours a day for treatment on weekdays as well as night times and holidays. In addition, the National Medical Center operated an emergency treatment center, and the military hospital opened its doors for treatment of emergency patients. Based on the "Emergency Medical Service Act," the Ministry of Health and Welfare has been establishing a basic emergency medical plan every five years since 2005.

---

17) Jeong Gi−hye (2017), Current Operation Status of Public Health Doctor System and Future Tasks, Korea Health Promotion Institute, Monthly Issue No.34

In 2002, the "Emergency Medical Service Act" was amended to provide the necessary financial resources for the improvement of the emergency medical system. In 2004, with the establishment of the National Emergency Department Information System (NEDIS), statistical data began to be generated for the establishment and execution of emergency medical policies.

Section 2

Current Status and Future Development of Healthcare Resources

1. Education, training, and professional development of health professionals

A. Education and training of physicians

From 1954 to 1960, the budget allocated for the public health sector accounted for only 0.97% of the total governmental budget on average, and the number of health professionals including doctors was insufficient. In 1945, with the health administration of the US military government taking over the police and sanitation administration during the Japanese colonial era, the state implemented a laissez−faire policy with a structure based on the division of labor; the state was only in charge of public health affairs and all medical services were delegated to the public sector.

With the outbreak of the Korean War in 1950, the foundation of national health care was hit hard, and due to the outbreak of infectious diseases at this time, the national health policy had no choice but to focus on all resources and activities in the field of quarantine and relief (Yoo Seung−heum [1990]). It was not until 1956 that the Public Health Clinic Act was enacted and promulgated, with the target of establishing public health centers in more than 500 locations across the country. However, it was only after the amendment of the Public Health Clinic Act in 1962 that a nationwide network of public health centers and regional centers was established (Korea Institute for Population and Health [now Korea Institute for Health and Social Affairs] [1987]).

After the liberation of Korea, national medical education began to take shape as the Japanese colonial system that governed major national and public medical institutions collapsed and an American−style medical system was introduced. The medical specialist system was introduced at this time, and in 1951, with the implementation of the National Permission System on Specialist Areas for Medical Service Providers in 1951, 10 specialist areas were determined under the National Medical Service Act. For 8 years from 1952, 1,427 permits for specialist areas were issued through the approval process of documentation review, and from 1960, permits were issued based on the examination system. In 1959, a national accreditation system for medical specialists was introduced, and in 1963, 510 interns and 924 residents were trained at 30 educational hospitals. This number indicates that the majority of medical school graduates aspired to become medical specialists.

Immediately after the liberation of the country, the supply of health professional manpower experienced a serious shortage. Although there was a slight increase until 1960, the brain drain phenomenon of medical personnel also increased. After the mid−1960s, Korean physicians went to the United States to settle down after completing their training, and nurses went to Germany or the United States to find employment, resulting in a manpower shortage in Korea. As for the number of health professionals, the number of physicians increased 1.8 times from 4,375 in 1949 to 7,765 in 1960, the number of dentists increased 1.9 times from 740 to 1,369, and the number of oriental medicine doctors increased 1.8 times from 1,657 to 2,922. The number of nurses also increased 3.1 times from 1,549 to 4,836, and the number of pharmacists increased 4.7 times from 1,003 to 4,696.

The first medical education institution in Korea was Gwanghyewon (House of Extended Grace), which opened in 1885, and in 1886, a year after its opening, the official medical education department was established for education in modern Western medicine. In 1897, 18 trained vaccinators graduated from the Vaccinator Training Institution. By 1910, six medical educational institutions had been established.

The national liberation triggered major changes in medical education. Medical education consisted of two years of premedical courses and four years of medical courses, and the university was in charge of the curriculum. The current established structure of a typical department of medicine in a college of medicine, which requires two years of basic medical science and two years of clinical medicine, was formed during this period. In 1952, the first national examination for a medical license was conducted. Before 1952, medical licenses were automatically awarded upon graduation from medical colleges and universities, but for the first time, a license was granted only to those who passed the national medical licensing examination from 1952. In 1959, the system of interns and residents was adopted in the medical curriculum. In 1962, the medical license examination system was abolished and the importance of medical schools increased. Until 1950, there were only six medical schools: the College of Medicine at Seoul National University, the College of Medicine at Kyungpook National University, Korea University, Yonsei University, Ewha Womans University, and Chonnam National University. However, 2 schools of medicine were established in the 1950s, 5 in the 1960s, 6 in the 1970s, 12 in the 1980s, and 10 after the 1990s. Since then, no more medical schools have been founded, resulting in 41 schools of medicine in total.

The reason that the foundation of new medical schools was concentrated in the 1980s and 1990s is because not only did the medical needs of the Korean public greatly increase following the economic growth and improved national income but also the demand for medical services increased rapidly due to the medical aid system and national medical insurance system being introduced in 1977, and so the government pushed ahead with a policy to increase the supply of doctors. With the continuous foundation of new medical schools, doctors' associations continued to raise the issue of the oversupply of doctors, fearing that the quality of doctors would deteriorate due to a shortage of teaching manpower and insufficient facilities at medical schools. Still, the government continued with a gradual increase in the establishment of new medical schools in preparation for increased demand for medical services.

The medical specialist system started from the institution of the 1951 National Permission System on Specialist Areas for Medical Service Providers. Specialized departments are defined in the provisions on the training and qualification of medical specialists in the Medical Service Act, and the National Permission System on Specialist Areas for Medical Service Providers started a provision from Article 4 of the National Medical Service Act: "A medical service provider cannot present or display its specialized department without the permission of the competent minister as determined by decree." Article 34 of the Enforcement Regulations of the National Medical Service Act stipulates 10 specialized departments: internal medicine, surgery, pediatrics, obstetrics and gynecology, ophthalmology, otolaryngology, dermatology and urology, psychiatry, orthopedics, and radiology. The training period required for qualification was set to five years, and an examination system for specialized departments was also implemented. Looking into the changes in the operation of the medical specialist system, the Council for Hospital Accreditation (now the Council for Graduate Medical Training), which is an organization under the Korean Hospital Association (KHA), the organization responsible for the operation of the medical specialist system, was established in March 1963 when the Ministry of Health and Social Affairs delegated the task of designating training hospitals to the Korea Medical Association. In 1967, the task of training hospital designation was transferred to the KHA, and since then, the KHA has been in charge of training hospital designation and quota allocation for the number of residents. The medical specialist qualification review committee was in operation from September 1969 to 1972. In February 1972, in accordance with the medical specialist training regulations, a medical training system review committee was established within the Ministry of Health and Social Affairs to review key matters of the medical training system, including training hospital standards, the number of trainees, the training curriculum and process, and other important matters. The name of the committee was changed to the Resident System Review Committee, with the change in the official name from trainee doctors to residents. Then, in September 1981, the provisions on this committee were deleted following the amendment of the Presidential Decree. In January 1973, the medical specialist qualification was accredited by the Minister of Health and Social Affairs based on a recommendation from the Central Association of Doctors, which was specified to be based on examination; therefore, the Korean Medical Association (KMA) took over the responsibility for the examination. In addition, as for the qualifying examination for medical specialists, it was assigned to the Korean Academy of Medical Sciences (previously the Association of Medical Sub−Committees) internally by the KMA, and for raising the standard of specialist expertise, the examination was directly commissioned to the Korean Academy of Medical Sciences from 2014. Examining the trends of examinees and those passing the medical specialist qualifying examination, the numbers increased by 6.68 times and 8.14 times, respectively, from 535 and 407 in 1976 to 3,573 and 3,313 in 2013 (Korea Medical Association [2013]). The number of medical specialists increased 29 times over 37 years from 2,805 in 1976 to 82,160 in 2013.

As the number of newly founded medical schools increased from the 1980s, concerns about the quality of medical school education and the oversupply of doctors began to rise. In the late 1990s, a number of studies were conducted on the trend in the supply and demand of doctors, and many reported on the issue of an oversupply of doctors. According to a report by a national policy research institute published in 1997, the quota for medical school admissions per 100,000 of national population was

7.8, which is much higher than in other developed countries. According to a report by the Korea Health Industry Development Institute published in 2000, it was predicted that in 2005, considering the number of medical doctors alone, there would be double the number of doctors specified by laws and, including Korean medicine doctors, the number of doctors would reach the level of countries with double Korea's national income, and after 2005 there would be an oversupply of doctors. In 2000, the Special Committee on Healthcare Service Development announced that the admission quota for newly founded medical schools was 40-50, indicating that the current state is not cost−effective considering the training cost of the doctors. In addition, due to problems such as a shortage of staff for teaching basic medical sciences, a shortage of training hospitals for clinical practice, and an oversupply considering the medical school admission quota per 100,000 of population of 7.1 (8.8 including Korean medicine doctors), a reduction of 20% in the admissions quota for medical schools was proposed as the most reasonable level for effective management (Special Committee on Healthcare Service Development [2000]). Based on the results of the meeting of the Special Committee on Healthcare Service Development, in August 2000, the Minister of Health and Welfare announced a healthcare service development plan to reduce the admission quota for medical schools by 10% with reference to the quota level in 2000 and to maintain the level by 2002.

In addition, before the Ministry of Education and Human Resources Development announced the "Master Plan for Introduction of a Medical and Dental Graduate School System" in January 2002, medical schools were operated based on an undergraduate course of two years of pre−medical courses and four years of medical courses. The Medical Graduate School (hereinafter MGS) is a course in which students who have obtained a bachelor's degree from a general undergraduate course are selected, receive doctor training for four years (4+4 system), and are awarded a master's degree in medicine. With the introduction of the MGS, the medical education system was run under the curriculums of 1) a college of medicine system, 2) an MGS system, or 3) an integrated system with a college of medicine system and an MGS system (hereinafter integrated MGS system). In 2003, two medical schools switched to the MGS system, and another two medical schools switched to the integrated MGS system, and since then, many universities have converted to MGS. Up to 2011, 27 colleges and 40 universities switched to MGS (integrated MGS). The remaining 13 universities have maintained their college of medicine systems. However, as of 2017, all but five MGSs had returned to the college of medicine system (Korea Medical Association Research Institute for Healthcare Policy [2014]).

B. Education and training of dentists

Dentistry education first began at Severance Hospital in 1922, and in 1946, the first formal educational institution for dentistry, the School of Dentistry at Seoul National University, was founded. Since dental colleges were established at Yonsei University and Kyunghee University in 1967, dentistry education has been delivered at 11 dental colleges and dental/medical graduate schools. In 1952, the first national examination for a dentistry qualification was conducted, and at this time, 24 students took the exam and 15 passed. In 2014, there were 28,123 registered dentists with licenses. Among them, 21,149 were employed in medical institutions.

In accordance with Article 55 of the Medical Service Act, the system for dental specialists is stipulated. In 1962, to open a dental clinic it was necessary to pass a qualifying examination conducted by the Korean Dental Association for the accredited specialized department. In October 1962, an attempt was made to implement a permission system for specialized departments based on an examination, but the examination was canceled due to nonattendance. In addition, the "Medical Specialist Training Regulations" were enacted and promulgated in 1972, specifying training—related matters in detail for medical and dental specialists. Meanwhile, in 1996, some dentists filed an unconstitutionality suit for not conducting dental specialist qualifying examinations. In response to the Constitutional Court's verdict of unconstitutionality in 1998, the Ministry of Health and Welfare enacted and implemented the "Regulations on the Training and Accreditation of Qualification for Dental Specialists" in 2003.

Trainee dentists undergo a training period of one year as an intern and three years as a resident. After the start of resident training in 2004, dentists sat the dental specialist qualifying examination for the first time in 2008. As a result, 221 dental specialists were qualified, and by 2014, 1,842 dental specialists were qualified. There are 10 specialized departments: oral and maxillofacial radiology, oral and maxillofacial surgery, preventive dentistry, oral medicine, oral pathology, prosthodontics, pediatric dentistry, periodontics, conservative dentistry, and orthodontics.

C. Education and training of Korean medicine doctors

Korean medicine was promoted in the late Joseon Dynasty, but after the signing of the Japan—Korea Treaty of 1876, it went into decline and Western medicine was introduced. The basic direction of healthcare policy came to revolve around Western medicine, resulting in the marginalization of Korean medicine. In the midst of these difficulties, Korean medicine doctors created a group called the General Association of Korean Medicine Doctors and made efforts to revive oriental medicine. However, in 1899, Korean medicine education was abolished from the formal curriculum, and eventually, even Korean medicine treatment was abolished from the formal treatment system in 1907. In particular, after the start of the Japanese colonial era, the status of Korean medicine doctors was also downgraded to medical students, leading to a natural decline (1913), and eventually, graduation of Korean medicine doctors was altogether blocked (1944). In response to the Western medicine—centered healthcare policy of Japan, the Korean medicine community responded by founding Korean medicine educational institutions, establishing Korean medicine organizations, holding promotional conferences, and publishing academic journals. However, these efforts were eventually overwhelmed by the fundamental policy of Japan trying to annihilate Korean medicine.

After the national liberation in 1945, the efforts of Korean medicine doctors to revive the national medicine continued. In the year of liberation, a Korean medicine organization called the Joseon Medical Association was established, and within a few years, the Oriental Medical Association was founded (1947), and the Oriental University for education in Korean medicine (1947) was also established, laying the groundwork for a revival of Korean medicine. These efforts led to activities to establish a Korean medicine practice system. Numerous Korean medicine doctors actively negotiated with lawmakers to introduce a Korean medicine practice system, and all their concerted efforts finally came to fruition. In 1951, during the Busan refugee period, the National Assembly passed a bill introducing a Korean medicine practice system 61 to 18, leading to the birth of a Korean medicine practice system in Korea. With the introduction of this system, studies of Korean medicine continued to develop. The foundation of academic development was consolidated during this period, such as the establishment of the Association of Oriental Medicine (1952), the launch of the Oriental Medicine Journal (1954), the promotion of Oriental Medicine School to Seoul Oriental Medicine University, and further development of Oriental Medicine University (1953). Although Oriental Medicine University faced a crisis due to the school reform ordinance in 1962, it was promoted to a six−year college of Korean medicine in 1964 through the efforts of the association and the activities of students and professors, and then merged with Kyung Hee University, continuing to operate today.

In response to the trend of modernization, the May 16th Military Government of Korea conducted the first total reform of the National Medical Service Act to the Medical Service Act (March 20, 1962) and attempted to abolish the Korean medicine practice system but encountered strong opposition from the Association of Korean Medicine Doctors. Therefore, the Medical Service Act underwent another amendment on December 13, 1963, resulting in a modernized form of the Korean medicine practice system. In other words, the Korean medicine education course was promoted to a six−year curriculum equivalent to the Western medicine education system, leading to stability in the curriculum. Based on the new change, Korean medicine doctors further enhanced and expanded various academic activities centered on the Association of Oriental Medicine, including hosting domestic and international academic conferences and conducting academic promotional projects.

In 1973, the 3rd Conference of the World Federation of Acupuncture−Moxibustion Societies, the first international academic event in the history of Korean medicine in Korea, was held in Seoul, hosted by the Association of Oriental Medicine, contributing to the reevaluation of Korean medicine. In 1973, the Medical Service Act was amended to allow the establishment of Korean medicine hospitals, and in 1975, the Medical Affairs 3 Department, an administrative body for Korean medicine, was established within the Ministry of Health and Social Affairs, facilitating the modernization of Korean medicine.

As government−funded projects, national policy projects related to Korean medicine continued to be developed, led by the government, such as research on setting standards for Korean herbal medicines, including the classification of diseases with comparisons of Korean and Western medicines, a survey on the current status of Korean medicine, and the publication of standard Korean medicine prescriptions.

In the 1980s, academic projects were developed to a mature stage, including correction of the name from oriental medicine to "Korean" medicine, supporting the domestic Korean medicine academic project of the World Health Organization, surveys on participation in Korean medicine health insurance, and other research projects. In addition, as the activities of the Society of Korean Medicine continued to be established, the number of divisions was increased to 19, and the number of Colleges of Korean Medicine was also increased to 11. Furthermore, with a number of recipients of master's degrees and PhDs in Korean medicine, a solid foundation for improving the quality of Korean medicine was established as one of the important pillars of treatment.

In 1988, national health insurance for Korean medicine was launched for the whole national population. Furthermore, to facilitate in−depth promotion of Korean medicine policy, the National Healthcare Policy Review Committee was formed to review the feasibility and validity of various long—term development projects, such as the establishment of a national Korean medicine hospital, the establishment of a specialized research institute, the institutionalization of Korean medicine health guidance, as well as a review of the feasibility of the Korean medicine specialist system, and these were reflected in policies in phases.

Since the 1970s, disputes over the preparation and prescription of Korean herbal medicines have continued, and this issue has been administratively pending since the National Assembly's additional resolution (December 17, 1975). Conflicts and tension between Korean medical doctors and pharmacists mounted prior to the amendment of the Pharmaceutical Affairs Act in March 1993. Then, the new government launched the Korean Medicine Development and Pharmaceutical Affairs Act Amendment Discussion Committee and collected opinions from academia for the improvement and development of Korean medicine institutionalization. In addition, the government and National Assembly established and announced a mid—to long—term development plan for the balanced development of Korean and Western medicine, while establishing the government—funded Korea Research Center of Oriental Medicine as a special corporation and subsequently expanding and rebuilding the Center as the Korea Institute of Oriental Medicine. The government has continued to improve the comprehensive Korean medicine development plan and various related institutions and systems and has taken promotional measures in order to enhance the contribution of Korean medicine to the public, such as the establishment of administrative organizations for Korean medicine and the institutionalization of the Korean medicine management system.

Currently, in Korea, there are 11 colleges of Korean medicine at Kyunghee University, Wonkwang University, Dongguk University, Gyeongsan University, Daejeon University, Kyungwon University, Sangji University, Semyeong University, Dongshin University, Dongeui University, Woosuk University in Jeonju, and the Graduate School of Korean Medicine at Pusan National University. There are more than 3,500 Korean medicine students in total. There are more than 20,000 practicing Korean medicine doctors who graduated from a college of Korean medicine. Research on Korean medicine has been led by these 12 colleges of Korean medicine and graduate schools of Korean medicine[18].

D. Education and training of nurses

The first nurse training school in Korea was the Bogu Nurse Training School, founded in 1903. In 1906, Severance Nursing School was founded, and in 1907, nursing education began to be provided at Daehan Hospital, which was the beginning of nursing education being officially implemented by the government. In July 1946, the existing training centers (nursing departments affiliated with hospitals and midwife training centers) were abolished and the education system was changed to include the Higher Education Center for Nursing. Eligibility for admission was a minimum of four years of middle school education, and the period for nursing education was unified at three years. At that time, there were 16 institutions for nursing education, including Red Cross Nursing High School, and the establishment of the Higher Education Center for Nursing was an opportunity to raise the level of nursing education to that of regular education. At the outbreak of the Korean War in 1950, most of the nursing education institutions were temporarily closed, but 13 schools reopened at the end of

---

18) History of Development of Korean Medicine—5. After the reform. [www.akom.org]

1951, and the number of enrolled nursing students in 1952 was 559. In addition, in 1951, the National Medical Service Act was enacted and promulgated, and the official name of nurses changed from "Ganho−bu" to "Ganho−won." The duty of nurses was defined as "nursing care or medical assistance for the sick or postpartum women," which formed the basis of the duties of modern nurses. From 1973, the qualifications for nursing school admission were unified as high school graduation, and in 1974, there was total reform of the system and the Higher Education Center for Nursing was closed.

In 1959, the Nursing School was established at the National Medical Center for junior−college−level courses. The admission criteria were high school graduation or higher, and the course was free. The nursing school, equivalent to a junior college, was officially named the Nursing School by the Education Act amended in 1962. The admission criteria were set to high school graduation, and a three−year course was operated. In March 1971, the course period for a nursing major was set to three years.

In January 1979, 36 nursing schools underwent reform to nursing colleges. For example, the Department of Nursing was established at the College of Medicine at Ewha Womans University in 1955; in 1957, the Department of Nursing at Severance Hospital was promoted to the Department of Nursing in the College of Medicine at Yonsei University; and in 1959, the Department of Nursing was founded at the College of Medicine of Seoul National University. In 1992, the Bachelor's Degree Examination for Self−Education system was introduced, and in 1996, special courses for nursing education (RN−BSN) were adopted. In 2006, the Credits Recognition System was established, and the number of four−year nursing colleges exceeded that of three−year nursing colleges. With the amendment of the Higher Education Act in May 2011, the "four−year nursing department" was introduced in junior colleges, and junior colleges that met the educational conditions stipulated in the Act were reviewed by the Korean Accreditation Board of Nursing Education, and when approved, they were entitled to run a bachelor's degree program (four−year system). Since 2012, the Ministry of Health and Welfare has been working with related organizations such as the Ministry of Education to promote the unification of the nursing college curriculum into a four−year system.

In January 2000, the name "nurse for each specialty" in Article 4 of the Medical Service Act was changed to "advanced practice nurse," and in October 2003, Articles 5 and 55 of the Enforcement Rule of the Medical Service Act increased the types of advanced practice nurse and applied more stringent standards for the qualification and specialization of advanced practice nurses to include public health, anesthesia, home care, psychiatric care, emergency care, industry care, infection control, elderly care, care for the critically ill, and hospice care. In November of the same year, a notice system for advanced practice nursing courses was established to prepare an institutional basis for the qualification of advanced practice nurses and the curriculum. Since 2004, a curriculum at the master's degree level has been in operation. In July 2006, the previous notice was accepted and enacted as separate additional rules under the Medical Service Act, "Rules on Accreditation of Advanced Practice Nurse Qualifications, etc.," and advanced practice nurses in the fields of pediatric care, oncology, and clinical practice were added. In addition, the advanced practice nurse qualifying examination has been conducted to promote excellent advanced practice nurses. The examination consists of a first stage (written) and a second stage (oral or clinical skills), and has been used to test advanced practice nurses since 2006.

E. Management of Health Professional Qualification

In the Health Professional Licensing Examination System, eligible applicants according to the provisions in the law need to pass a national examination, and any possible disqualifying factors are checked. Finally, the license is granted by the Minister of Health and Welfare. That is, in the licensing examination system, comprehensive capabilities required in clinical practice such as professional knowledge, clinical skills, attitude, and ethics are assessed, and only those who have satisfied the criteria specified by the applicable laws are granted the exclusive right to treat disease and conduct health promotion for the Korean population.

The Health Professional Licensing Examination has been administered by the Public Health Examination Division of the Ministry of Health and Social Affairs for about 40 years since the commencement of the first examination system for doctors, dentists, and Korean medicine doctors in 1952. In October 1986, the Ministry of Health and Social Affairs established the Medical Service Management Committee as a ministerial advisory body to review major healthcare policy matters, such as healthcare system improvement, health professional manpower supply plans, and the management of doctors' national examination. Further, it conducted institutional improvement of the medical licensing examination. In 1992, the Korea Medical Licensing Examination Institute was established as a type of private foundation, and for medical licensing examinations only, the examination management was commissioned to a private evaluation organization.

The validity and reliability of the medical licensing examination were recognized, but there was the issue of the impartiality of the examination for Korean medicine preparation. Therefore, for the sake of a new setting and the transfer of the organization of all health professional licensing examinations such as Korean medicine doctors, dentists, pharmacists, and nurses, the existing Korea Medical Licensing Examination Institute was reformed and expanded into the Korea Health Professional Licensing Examination Institute (hereinafter KHPLEI) in 1998. Since the end of 2014, the national examinations for 24 occupations and 28 departments that include health professionals have been conducted and managed by the KHPLEI.

The Ministry of Health and Welfare approved and announced the introduction of a clinical skills test for physicians in June 2006 based on the 1st Master Plan for Health Professional Development (2006–2010). The purpose was to improve healthcare services for the public by enhancing the quality of health professionals.

At the end of September 2009, a clinical skills test was introduced for the first time in Asia and the third time in the world for the sake of medical licensing examination. It evaluates the clinical skills of doctors and contributes to the provision of improved healthcare services to the public. Furthermore, it has served as a role model for the expansion of clinical skills tests in other occupations and the introduction of such tests for other national examinations in Asia.

In addition, from 2011, in order to improve the standard of the National Health Professional Licensing Examination, a computerized test was introduced that simulates clinical settings through multimedia such as videos. This has been actively promoted over paper—based exams, so that the performance of health professionals in clinical settings can fully benefit from the new type of test.

To provide improved healthcare services to the public by maintaining the professional standard of healthcare personnel, health professionals were required to complete continuing education for at least eight hours every year after acquiring their license. However, the management system has been poor, and there has been a low completion rate of the mandatory continuing education and a lack of information on the current employment status of licensed health professionals. To address these problems, in July 2009, the Ministry of Health and Welfare formed a consultative body with the participation of the government, medical institutions, and academics from the relevant research fields to prepare a follow−up management system for licensees in health professions.

The License Registration System, which has been implemented since April 2012 following the amendment of the Medical Service Act in April 2011, requires that health professionals complete continuing education every year and report their current situation including their employment status every three years. After the implementation of the system, bulk registration (until April 2013) was conducted for one year, and thereafter, the system was reformed into a periodic registration system in which reports are made every three years from the license grant date for new license holders and from the date of the last license report for existing license holders. In addition, medical service technicians also conducted bulk registration from January to November 2015 following the implementation of the License Registration System in November 2014 according to the amendment of the Medical Service Technicians, etc. Act in November 2011.

Following these reforms, through the License Registration System, the employment status of health professionals has been identified to prepare basic reference statistics for health professional supply and demand policies, and continuing education has been stringently managed, thereby contributing to the provision of improved healthcare services to the public and the creation of a safe healthcare environment[19].

---

19) Ministry of Health and Welfare, 『70 Years of History in Health and Welfare』 Vol. 2 Healthcare Service, 2016.

Section 3

Changes in Health Care Organizations and the Present

1. Changes in the Government Organization Centered on the Ministry of Health and Welfare

A. Changes in the Organization of the Ministry of Health and Welfare

The Ministry of Health and Welfare, formerly called the Ministry of Health and Social Affairs, was launched by merging the Ministry of Health and the Ministry of Social Affairs in 1955 as a system consisting of 22 departments in six bureaus. Since then, the organization of the Ministry of Welfare has been increased to four offices, three bureaus, 15 department officers, and 65 departments by 2020. The number of health care─related departments in the administrative organization has increased: 1955 (22 departments 56) → 1970 (12 departments) → 1980 (28 departments) → 1990 (29 departments) → 2003 (26 departments) → 2010 (65 departments).

The changes in the names of health care─related government agencies and departments by era are as follows[20].

---

20) Ministry of Health and Social Affairs 1955─1994. [www.mohw.go.kr]

· Establishment of Ministry of Social Affairs (1948): In charge of affairs associated with health, welfare, labor, housing, and women

· Establishment of the Ministry of Health (1949): In charge of affairs associated with public health, sanitation, regulations, quarantine, and agreements

· Merging into the Ministry of Health and Social Affairs (1955): In charge of affairs associated with duties, quarantine, health, sanitation, medicine, relief, assistance, welfare, housing, women, and labor

· Reorganization into the Ministry of Health and Welfare (1994): In charge of affairs associated with health and hygiene, quarantine, regulations, agreements, livelihood protection, support for self-reliance, women's welfare, children (excluding infant care), the elderly, the disabled, and social security

· Reorganization into the Ministry for Health, Welfare and Family Affairs (February 2008): In charge of affairs associated with health hygiene, quarantine, regulations, agreements, livelihood protection, support for self-reliance, social security, children (including infant care), youth, the elderly, the disabled, and families

· Reorganization into the Ministry of Health and Welfare (March 2010): In charge of the affairs related to health and welfare policies, with the youth and family-associated functions transferred to the Ministry of Gender Equality and Family

B. Establishment of Major Institutions under the Ministry of Health and Welfare

In 1998, the Ministry of Food and Drug Safety was established as an independent organization under the Ministry of Health and Welfare in order to respond to the growing public awareness and interest in "food." With the National Toxicology Research Institute and six regional offices (Seoul/Busan/Gyeongin/Daegu/Gwangju/Daejeon) as affiliated organizations, it was launched with a capacity of 776 people (as of 2011, the capacity was 1,454). In 2010, the safety management of alcoholic beverages, which had been managed by the National Tax Service, was transferred to the Food and Drug Administration in charge of food and drug safety management.

When the government was first established, affairs associated with food and drugs were under the jurisdiction of the Ministry of Health. Then, in 1994, it was reorganized as the Food Bureau to ensure food safety. In 1995, the government led by President Kim Young−sam began to consider the establishment of the Food and Drug Administration. In April 1996, the Food and Drug Safety Headquarters was established as an independent organization under the Ministry of Health and Welfare in order to ensure and unify a professional and comprehensive safety management system for illegal and harmful foods and medicines. Since the management system was still at a basic level, there was a need for establishing a dedicated body, considering that food and drug safety were the basis of public health. Prior to the inauguration of President Kim Dae−jung, the transition team presented a basic model of the Food and Drug Administration modeled after the US FDA, stressing the need for such promotion by saying, "Even in developed countries, there is a trend to change the food management task from the agriculture and forestry department to the health department or to establish a dedicated department in order to protect the public health." On February 28, 1998, the Food and Drug Administration was established to strengthen the safety management function for food and drugs. In addition to authority and status, the government led by President Roh Moo−hyun benchmarked the FDA in order to strengthen the "speed, efficiency, and accountability" of the organization. In order to improve the problem that the technical administration and the technical review organization were divided, failing to cooperate, it was decided to reorganize it into a headquarters/team system, with reference to the function−integrated center system. However, despite these efforts, the "Korean version of the FDA" did not come to life as a wide range of food−related tasks, from production, manufacturing, and consumption, were dispersed among the Ministry of Welfare, the Ministry of Oceans and Fisheries, and the Ministry of Agriculture and Forestry, failing to achieve unification.

In 2013, under the government of President Park Geun−hye, it was promoted as the Ministry of Food and Drug Safety under the Prime Minister due to its elevated status. This was to meet the aim of "unifying the food safety management," and the budget and manpower increased accordingly[21].

The Korea Centers for Disease Control and Prevention (KCDC) started in 2003 with the abolition of the National Institute of Health and the establishment of the Korea Centers for Disease Control and Prevention for a more systematic approach to disease management. Looking into its origin in more detail, the Korea Centers for Disease Control and Prevention originated as the Sanitation Bureau, established by the edict of King Gojong in 1894. After that, based on the health center training center established in 1935, after liberation in 1945, these institutions were renamed the Joseon Quarantine Research Institute and the National Chemical Research Institute[22]. On December 16, 1963, the National Institute of Health was established by merging the National Quarantine Research Institute, the National Chemical Research Institute, the National Institute of Health, and the National Institute of Herbal Medicine, which had been established and operated as independent institutions.

In 1999, the Department of Infectious Disease Control was established within the National Institute of Health, which was expanded and reorganized to respond to infectious diseases in 2004. At the time of the SARS outbreak in 2003, the departments in charge of infectious diseases and quarantine consisted of only two to three people from the National Institute of Health under the Ministry of Health and Welfare. Accordingly, the necessity of establishing an organization for systematic countermeasures against infectious diseases was highlighted. Commissioner Jeong Eun−kyung said, "KCDC was created during an evaluation meeting with former President Roh Moo−hyun after overcoming SARS." Subsequently, the Centers for Disease Control and Prevention (KCDC) were established by modeling after the Centers for Disease Control and Prevention (CDC).

With the global pandemic of COVID−19 in 2020 and the large−scale infections in Korea, there was a pressing need to strengthen the quarantine capacity of the government. On September 12, 2020, it was promoted to the Korea Disease Control and Prevention Agency. An organization started as a team of two to three people

---

21) Ministry of Food and Drug Safety. [ko.wikipedia.org]

22) Korea Centers for Disease Control and Prevention. [www.cdc.go.kr]

finally became an agency after serving as a center. Quarantine stations are also affiliated with the Korea Disease Control and Prevention Agency, which acts as the only independent organization that comprehensively manages infectious diseases that can be introduced or developed from inside or outside the country[23].

Looking at the progress of the health insurance management and operation system in relation to the National Health Insurance, the workplace medical insurance, which was launched on July 1, 1977, based on the Medical Insurance Act enacted in 1963 and amended in 1976, for employers with 500 or more employees, was the beginning of the health insurance system in Korea[24].

Meanwhile, the Medical Insurance Management Corporation, established by the "Medical Insurance Act for Government and Private School Employees" enacted in 1977 and its enforcement decree, started providing medical insurance benefits for government and private school employees, as well as their dependents, in January 1979. It covered 4.94 million people by the end of 1997.

In addition, from January 1988, medical insurance began to be applied to residents of rural and fishing villages. From July 1989, insurance benefits were also provided to the self−employed in urban areas, achieving national health insurance coverage for the first time in 12 years since the introduction of medical insurance.

As of July 1989, it was divided into three parts: medical insurance for employees, medical insurance for government and private school employees, and regional medical insurance. All those who applied for voluntary regional medical insurance and occupational medical insurance before 1987 were covered by regional medical insurance[25].

Korea's health (medical) insurance system, which started with low premiums and low wages for the prompt launch of medical insurance at the end of 1977, fell into a whirlpool of great upheaval with the launch of the National Health Insurance Service on October 1, 1998, based on the National Medical Insurance Act, which aimed at integrating regional medical insurance into the medical insurance for government and private school employees under the management of the Medical Insurance Service, passed by the National Assembly.

In January 1999, the "National Health Insurance Act" was passed by the National Assembly with the aim of removing structural barriers to financial management by cooperatives, securing insurance finances at the national level and guaranteeing an appropriate level of medical service based on this. Based on this, on July 1, 2000, the Medical Insurance Service and 139 employee health insurance programs were merged, and the National Health Insurance Service, a single insurance program covering the entire nation, was launched to achieve organizational integration. After one delay, the financial integration of health insurance was achieved on July 1, 2003, putting an end to the process of complete integration of health insurance in Korea, which took about five years.

---

23) With respect to COVID−19, "the Central Administrative Agency Organization and the Disease Control System of Korea" [blog.naver.com]

24) Moon Il−bong (2011), A Study on the Improvement Plan of CT Insurance Fee According to the Technological Development of CT, Chonnam National University Graduate School, August 2011.

25) Encyclopedia of Korean Culture (National Health Service): http://encykorea.aks.ac.kr/Contents/Item/E0043194

With the integration of health insurance in 2000, the Health Insurance Review and Assessment (HIRA) Service began to deal with the medical expense review, which was previously managed by the Medical Insurance Association, reflecting the opinion of the health care community that the medical expense review organization was independent. Since then, there have been criticisms from the medical community that the HIRA is overly regulating along with the positive evaluation that it is evaluating the appropriateness of the quality of medical care.

The Korea Health Industry Development Institute was established in 1998 when the Korea Institute of Health Services Management and the Food and Drug Research Institute merged. At that time, the Korea Institute of Health Services Management was a research institute that developed into a public—private joint research institute from a hospital research institute affiliated with Seoul National University Hospital. After being reorganized into the Korea Health Industry Development Institute, the contribution of the private sector to the Korea Medical Management Research Institute was returned to the Korea Hospital Association (KHA) and the Korean Medical Association (KMA), respectively. Based on the contributions, the two institutions are operated as the Korean Institute of Hospital Management (KHA, a foundation) and the Research Institute for Healthcare Policy (KMA, a department at KMA), respectively.

In 1992, to accommodate the private sector—led demands from the health care and medical communities, the Korea Health Personnel Licensing Examination Institute was established as a foundation. Since 2010, it has also been in charge of licensing examinations for care workers and nurse assistants.

In accordance with Article 58 of the Medical Service Act, the Korea Institute for Healthcare Accreditation is in charge of granting accreditation, which means that a medical institution has achieved patient safety and an appropriate level of quality in the process of providing all medical services (Kim Young—man, 2012)[26]. In the early days of the Korean Hospital Standardization Program (currently, hospital accreditation evaluation), it was conducted by the Korea Hospital Association in relation to health care quality management. Since 2004, the Korea Health Industry Development Institute has been in charge of compulsory evaluation, and in 2010, the Institute for Evaluation and Certification of Medical Institutions was established, with a separate foundation being established and operated to autonomously manage patient safety and health care quality (Lee Kyu—sik, 2012)[27].

26) Kim Young—man (2012), A Study on the Introduction of the Laboratory Accreditation System for Safety Management.

27) Lee Kyu—sik (2012), Changes in the Socio—economic Environment and the Direction of Health Care Policy, Research Institute for Healthcare Policy of the Korea Medical Association, 2012.

2. Establishment and Development of Health Care-related Organizations

A. Korea Hospital Association

The latter half of the 1950s was an era when the size of private hospitals and small and medium−sized hospitals underwent expansion and large general hospitals appeared. Therefore, business management problems emerged little by little, and a unified voice representing the hospital was needed to solve these problems. The Korean Hospital Association (KHA) was established in 1959 with the approval of the Ministry of Health and Social Affairs, as the government agreed that such an organization was necessary for the smooth implementation of national medical policies.

In 1980, KHA selected the Korean Hospital Standardization Program as a priority. The Korea Hospital Association established a policy to review patient treatment standards, safety management and maintenance, organizational function and management, infection prevention measures, quality control of pathology tests, etc. As a result, achievements such as the establishment of medical ethics and the improvement in the quality of patient care were expected. The first hospital standardization survey was conducted in 1981. As a result of conducting a survey of 110 training hospitals across the country, they were experiencing great difficulties in securing a workforce of doctors in general. Areas to be improved and supplemented, such as hospital infection control and medical social work, were revealed. The second survey was carried out based on the project of the previous year by conducting a survey of 135 training hospitals across the country. The overall score of the second survey was lower compared to the previous year, as the survey itself was changed from a guidance assessment to a performance−based assessment.

In 1986, negotiations for the Uruguay Round officially started. Finally, in January 1994, a meeting on the opening of the health care service market was held by the Ministry of Health and Social Affairs. This meeting was aimed at discussing the anticipated problems and countermeasures following the opening of the market. Major issues in the fields associated with the opening of the market and market entry prediction models were analyzed, and health care service−related laws and regulations of Korea and foreign countries were compared. The KHA emphasized that in order to increase competitiveness in the global market, it was necessary for Korean hospitals to improve their level of hospital treatments and services while the government provided support, such as the realization of medical insurance fees and the improvement of unreasonable hospital−related taxation.

B. Korean Academy of Medical Sciences

The first society established in Korea was the Joseon Neuropsychiatric Association, which was organized immediately after the liberation of Korea in September 1945, followed by a variety of subspecialty.

In 1966, the Korean Institute of Medical Science, the predecessor of the Korean Academy of Medical Sciences, was established. In April 1967, the KMA recognized the Korean Institute of Medical Science as the official body of the KMA. In 1974, the activities of the Korean Institute of Medical Science were defined as the official activities of the Korean Medical Association. Currently, the Korean Academy of Medical Sciences is an organization that supports academic activities as a council of academic divisions under KMA.

The institute strived to plan and carry out its own responsibilities and functions until the late 1980s. The examination of specialists was transferred from the National Institute of Health to KMA, and work related to specialist education and training was strengthened, and developments were made, such as publishing a collection of abstracts on Korean medicine in English.

In 1987, the Korean Institute of Medical Science was renamed the Korean Academy of Medical Sciences. From 1988 to 1994, the Korean Academy of Medical Sciences promoted basic medicine promotion projects, international exchange projects, academic journal publication projects, and medical education revitalization projects, thereby promoting the development of various societies in the health care and medical community. Representative projects included the publication of training courses for hospital openings, workshops, the publication of medical glossaries, the hosting of international conferences, and joint research projects between Korea and the United States in the field of cancer.

A fundamental challenge arose in the 1990s: identifying the perspective from which the subdivided academic societies should be dealt with. In order to address this problem, research to establish a new classification system, totally different from the existing member classification, was carried out. First, the systems in Japan, the United States, and Europe having a structure similar to that of the Korean Academy of Medical Sciences were analyzed, inferring the correlation between the parent society and the sub−society, as well as the specialized society. Through this research project, the classification system of the academic societies was established, and the classification of members became clearer, laying the foundation for the current member society accreditation review and academic activity evaluation. From 2003, the revised regular report was applied and the results were evaluated after receiving submissions from member societies[28].

C. Korean National Tuberculosis Association

The first modern tuberculosis care center in Korea was established in 1928 by a Canadian missionary doctor, Sherwood Hall. He took care of many patients by disseminating correct tuberculosis knowledge and introducing the latest equipment and started the anti−tuberculosis campaign by issuing Korea's first Christmas seals in Korea, in 1932.

Although the Korean War was a tragedy, it also provided an opportunity to develop tuberculosis pathology in Korea by rapidly introducing the latest medicines from the United States and advanced countries. In addition, the desperate tuberculosis situation served as an opportunity to gather people associated with tuberculosis from all over the country to organize a nationwide private organization. At that time, the Korean Tuberculosis Prevention Association, the Korean Tuberculosis Association, and the Tuberculosis Countermeasure Committee were dissolved, and a single civilian anti−tuberculosis organization was launched in 1953. The donation from the American−Korean Foundation was the only source of funding right after the organization was founded, but the Korean National Tuberculosis

---

28) 50 Years of the Korean Academy of Medical Sciences. [www.kams.or.kr]

Association then started issuing Christmas seals while raising awareness of tuberculosis prevention with banners, posters, and newspaper advertisements.

As the projects expanded and developed rapidly in the 1960s during the economic growth period, problems arose due to the lack of tuberculosis management skills and a shortage in the workforce at public health centers. Accordingly, the association hired and trained a workforce to be deployed to public health centers and then dispatched them to 189 public health centers nationwide as tuberculosis control officers, who took charge of the tuberculosis management project at public health centers.

In the 1990s, domestic training by inviting foreign experts and the dispatch of Korean experts abroad increased to broaden and strengthen international exchange. In 1995, the Tuberculosis Research Center was designated as a WHO partner institution to conduct research, training, and advisory roles on tuberculosis.

In 2000, the Tuberculosis Surveillance Center was opened at the Tuberculosis Research Center, and a surveillance system enabling real−time tuberculosis information on the Internet was established. This facilitated the analysis of tuberculosis outbreaks, the construction of databases, the identification of trends, the identification of the current status of tuberculosis and the search for patients. The tuberculosis information monitoring system was then transferred to the Korea Centers for Disease Control and Prevention in 2007 and expanded to an integrated tuberculosis information management system (TBnet) in 2010.

D. Korea Association of Health Promotion

Korea suffered from many infectious diseases along with social chaos after the 8.15 liberation. Infectious diseases such as cholera, smallpox, and malaria have left many people suffering and taking their lives. Hepatic distoma and parasitic infections were also commonly found during this period. In order to cure these parasite−related diseases, the Korean Association for Parasite Eradication was established in 1964. In 1969, the association was designated as an institution to conduct group testing for elementary, middle, and high school students by the Ministry of Education and contributed to reducing the parasite infection rate from over 80% to 2% by carrying out the "National Parasite Eradication Project"[29].

As a result of the national efforts to manage parasites, the parasite infection rate, which exceeded 80% in the early days of establishment, began to decrease sharply in the 1980s, but chronic diseases due to economic growth and changes in diet emerged as a new health problem. In order to more effectively use the technology, workforce, and facilities accumulated through the parasite projects, the Korean Association for Parasite Eradication established the Korea Association of Health Promotion in 1982, setting a new goal to contribute to the promotion of public health through early detection and prevention of non−communicable chronic diseases. In 1986, the two associations were merged as the focus of the association was shifted to health promotion projects, and the name was changed to the Korea Association of Health Promotion. The association further revitalized health screenings, surveys, and health

---

29) [Health & Beauty] News from the "Korea Association of Health Promotion," which has been protecting public health for 52 years. [www.donga.com]

education projects.

In the 21st century, the Korea Association of Health Promotion signed agreements with various social groups to activate the national health checkup project, provided high−quality health care services in response to the rapidly changing health care environment, and operated health counseling centers in 15 branches to support health promotion programs for local residents. In addition, international cooperation began to take off in earnest, followed by a series of health care projects in developing countries such as Mongolia, Cambodia, and Sudan. Starting with the parasite management project in China in 1995, the association has been carrying out projects in eight countries based on its experience in eradicating parasites in Korea. In particular, in Laos and Cambodia, the association supported the health promotion of residents through parasite management projects and surveys on the rate of parasite infection. In Mongolia, Indonesia, and Myanmar, projects targeting students, such as education on healthy living practices and smoking prevention education for children, were conducted.

With an increase in life expectancy, "living healthy for a long time" has emerged as a major topic. Accordingly, the association has focused on its role as a medical institution specializing in health promotion, introducing the latest examination equipment such as MRI, MDCT, and ultrasound equipment. New test items, such as genetic tests, and new screening programs, such as cancer screening, are being developed and implemented.

E. Planned Parenthood Federation of Korea

The Korean family planning movement changed in earnest when the Planned Parenthood Federation of Korea was founded in 1961. Afterwards, it was renamed and operated as the Korea Family Health and Welfare Association (February 1999–November 2005) in 1999 and the Korea Population, Health and Welfare Association in 2005, respectively[30].

Family planning was promoted through the government−led public−private cooperative method, in which the Ministry of Health and Social Affairs established a division of labor with private organizations such as the Planned Parenthood Federation of Korea. In Korea, with no experience in national family planning, public−private partnership was the key to the success of the project, and it was the Planned Parenthood Federation of Korea that led the cooperation. In various pilot research projects, the association served as a bridge with the academic community and served as a bridge for the academic community to participate in various councils to provide academic support.

Unlike the maternal and child health project, which was linked to government projects during the population growth suppression policy period, the maternal and child health project focused on improving the quality of the population during the population quality improvement policy period. In particular, since the 1990s, the scope of the maternal and child health project has included not only pregnant women and infants, but also unmarried women and adolescents who need preparation for motherhood. Provision of the benefits to the vulnerable was carried out in association

---

30) Sam−Sik Lee, Study on the 50 Years of Population Policy.

with public health centers and private organizations such as the Korean Family Health and Welfare Association. Through sex education for adolescents, a program was developed to link the prevention of sexually transmitted infections and HIV/AID. Education and public relations were focused on adolescent sexual problems, gender imbalance, and artificial abortions, away from family planning.

In the 21st century, a serious population problem and a very low fertility problem emerged as social problems, which became more apparent with the social advancement of women. After the Korean Economic Crisis in 1997, there has been an increased tendency to postpone marriage, stay single, or have fewer children. As the total fertility rate, which had been stably maintained between 1.5 and 1.7 in the mid−1980s, decreased to 1.5 for the first time in 1998, it showed a further downward trend to 1.08 in 2005. Accordingly, responses to the aging population and low fertility began in earnest with the enactment of the Framework Act on Low Birth Rate in an Aging Society in 2005, during the administration of President Roh Moo−hyun.

The association also changed the focus of its projects from childbirth suppression to encouragement and encouraged childbirth by installing breastfeeding and milking rooms and introducing support for infertile couples.

In the 21st century, international exchange was also active. The aid projects for the Chinese Korean Autonomous Prefecture started, and overseas exchange projects with Vietnam and China progressed even further. In 2013, as a result of carrying out population projects for the past 50 years, it was certified as a "Health Promoting Hospital" by the World Health Organization (WHO).

F. Korean Medical Association

Immediately after the liberation of Korea on August 15, there were several societies, such as the "Founding Medical Association," organized mainly by medical practitioners, and the "Joseon Medical Research Society" and the "Joseon Medical Association," organized by medical school professors, causing confusion. These organizations came together on May 10, 1947, by launching the nationwide "Joseon Medical Association." Through the resolution of the extraordinary general meeting on September 21, 1948, right after the establishment of the government, the name was changed to the "Korea Medical Association Organization." KMA has achieved various achievements, including holding academic conferences and publishing the Journal of the Korean Medical Association. A representative achievement achieved with respect to the government in the early days of reconstruction was the independence of the Ministry of Health from the Ministry of Social Affairs.

KMA has successfully established itself as an "organization with the people" rather than an "organization only for doctors" by conducting various public projects, such as the hepatitis eradication campaign in 1981, the Life Sayer and medical information card distribution in 1982, the food poisoning prevention campaign in 1983, the anti−smoking campaign in 1985, and the campaign to prevent fetal sex discrimination in 1995. KMA changed its name from "Korea Medical Association" to "Korean Medical Association" for the first time in 47 years, as the articles of association were revised following the decision at the general meeting of KMA in April 1995.

On February 27, 1997, the Medical Association confirmed and promulgated the "Doctors' Ethics Declaration." On April 12, 1997, the "Code of Ethics for Doctors" was enacted and promulgated, and on November 15, 2001, the finalized "Guidelines for Doctors' Ethics" were officially proclaimed on April 19, in commemoration of the 93rd anniversary of KMA. Since 1908, when Korea's first medical association, the Doctors Research Association, was established, the medical community has undergone many numerous changes. These changes in the medical community have been made in conjunction with changes in society as a whole. Recently, there have been a number of cases where the professional interests of doctors and social demands collide. Since these problems often arise in the absence of communication with society, it is necessary for a medical association to secure many channels to communicate smoothly with society. Such a channel cannot be secured all of a sudden when the necessity arises as a matter directly related to the interests of the parties occur. Therefore, it is necessary to listen to the needs of society on a regular basis and make efforts to gain recognition as a responsible member of society through various activities.

Section 4

Aspects of the Development of Changes in the Health Insurance System

1. Birth and Early Development of the Medical Insurance System

The medical insurance system was born by reflecting the views of the people and those who led the country at the time to build a new national system after the liberation and the Korean War in the hopes of achieving stability and prosperity in people's lives.

Korea started including health and medical welfare during social welfare in the 5.16 military government period (May 1961–December 1963) (Moon Byung–ju, 2005)[31]. The Ministry of Health and Social Affairs presented a plan for the medical insurance project in the 1961 supplementary budget (draft). In February 1963, the draft of the "Medical Insurance Act" was submitted by the Medical Insurance Group through the "First Five–Year Economic Development Plan (1962–1966)". Where, compulsory medical insurance was stipulated for workers in workplaces with 500 or more employees (Son Jun–gyu, 1981)[32]. The compulsory application for workplaces with 500 or more employees was modified to a voluntary application for workplaces with 300 or more employees. During the construction deliberation process for the amendment bill of the Ministry of Health and Social Affairs and the Culture and Society Committee, the voluntary application was confirmed. Accordingly, in December 1963, the regulation on the compulsory collection of GW fees was deleted and the "Medical Insurance Act" was enacted.

Changes in the political situation, such as North Korea's publicity for free health care and the reformation in 1972, also contributed to the introduction of the medical insurance system. In September 1976, the Ministry of Health and Social Affairs announced the "Measures to Expand Medical Benefits for the Improvement of Public Health" (the "Expansion Plan"), which had been studied by the Social Security Committee.95) The Medical Insurance Act, which aimed at implementing compulsory application, was promulgated in December 1976 and came into effect in July 1977. The main contents of the "Medical Insurance Act" are as follows.

---

31) Moon Byung–ju (2005), Industrial Relations and the Character of the Korean Welfare System: A Reinterpretation of the Industrialization Period, Korean Political Science Review 39(5):153–177.

32) Son Jun–gyu (1981), A Study on the Welfare Policy Decision Process in Korea, Seoul National University Doctoral Dissertation.

Compulsory and voluntary applications shall be applied in parallel, but the scope of compulsory application will be expanded in stages, from workplaces of a certain size or larger. The insurants are divided into type 1 insurants (workers at the workplace) and type 2 insurants (general residents and persons other than type 1). The insurer manages and operates the insurance business through the cooperatives, and the government supervises the cooperatives. Type 1 cooperatives consist of workers and employers at the workplace, and type 2 cooperatives consist of local residents based on administrative district units.

Although the government led and decided on the introduction of the medical insurance system, the opinions of companies and the medical community were also taken into account. However, the interests of workers were not reflected enough as they were not allowed to form unions at that time. The Korea Medical Association (the Korean Medical Association after May 1995) was very interested in insurance fees and insurance drug prices, and invited representatives of the medical community to the insurance review body. The Federation of Korean Industries took a positive stance on the introduction of the system.

When it was decided to implement medical insurance in the form of a cooperative in July 1977, it became important to promptly establish a medical insurance cooperative. The Ministry of Health and Social Affairs delivered the list of workplaces that were subject to the application of medical insurance to the Medical Insurance Council. The council worked closely with economic organizations such as the Federation of Korean Industries, the Korea Chamber of Commerce and Industry, and the Korea Enterprises Federation to establish the cooperatives.

It was as important to secure health care institutions (inpatient care institutions) along with the establishment of medical insurance cooperatives. However, insurance contracts with health care institutions did not go smoothly. Health care institutions were skeptical of health insurance as the medical treatment fee set by the government were low. The Ministry of Health and Social Affairs requested cooperation from KHA and KMA in July 1977. They were persuaded that the government−announced medical treatment fee had been lowered from the conventional medical treatment fee in the market, but the medical treatment income would not fall with the guaranteed payment of insurance medical expenses, an increased number of patients, and an increased bed occupancy rate. It was also pointed out that medical insurance would not put much pressure on the management of health care institutions as it only covered less than 10% of the population. As a result, at the end of December 1977, there were an average of about 50 medical institutions designated by medical insurance per cooperative, with no great difficulty for medical insurance policyholders in using medical institutions. However, at the beginning of the implementation, some hospitals received an additional 50% of the cost of treatment in the name of "special treatment." In addition, there were cases in which patients did not disclose that they were medical insurance policyholders or avoided using designated medical institutions for fear that hospitals would discriminate against patients with medical insurance. When medical insurance was first implemented for workplaces employing 500 or more employees, the Federation of Korean Industries (FKI) actively cooperated. Beyond its role as a stakeholder, FKI had a significant impact on medical insurance operations and policymaking for nearly 20 years, until health insurance was fully integrated in July 2000. Close cooperation between the government and the business community has contributed to the successful establishment of health insurance.

In July 1979, it was expanded to workplaces with 300 or more employees, and in January 1981, it was expanded to workplaces with 100 or more employees.

In January 1983, two years after it was applied to workplaces with 100 or more employees in January 1981, it was expanded to workplaces with 16 or more employees. With the amendment of the Enforcement Decree in December 1982, it became mandatory for workplaces with 16 or more employees, and workplaces with five or more employees could subscribe to the service voluntarily.

In January 1988, medical insurance was expanded to residents of rural areas, and in July 1988, the government revised the Enforcement Decree and expanded it to businesses with five or more employees. Since workplaces with five or more employees were subject to voluntary application, most of them were not covered by medical insurance. However, there was a difficult situation. In January 1988, when medical insurance was implemented in rural areas, workers in workplaces with five or more but less than 16 employees having an address in rural areas (gun areas) were subject to the compulsory application of regional medical insurance. The workers of small businesses, who had to pay insurance premiums as regional medical insurance subscribers, hoped to be incorporated into the employee medical insurance program as soon as possible. However, employers of small businesses were reluctant to join the employee medical insurance program due to the high premiums. Although the burden on employers of small businesses was large, the government has decided to reduce the burden on employees and provide medical insurance benefits to more people.

According to the government's decision, when the application was expanded to workplaces with five or more employees, some employers avoided medical insurance as they could not bear the burden. Nevertheless, the number of workplaces with five or more but less than 16 employees increased by 41% from 37,730 at the end of 1987 to 53,371 at the end of 1988 (Medical Insurance Association [1997]).

As compulsory medical insurance coverage expanded to businesses with five or more employees, the expansion of medical insurance for businesses with fewer than five employees emerged as an important policy issue. As medical insurance expanded to rural areas in 1988 and urban areas in 1989, workers in these small businesses had to pay insurance premiums as regional medical insurance subscribers. It was necessary to solve the problem of large differences in insurance premiums depending on whether they worked for workplaces with five or more employees or workplaces with fewer than five employees, despite being paid the same amount at work.

With the integration of medical insurance in July 2000, the application of employee medical insurance to small businesses with fewer than five employees were taken into consideration. The National Health Insurance Act, amended in December 2000, expanded the scope of employee medical insurance to workplaces with one or more employees. The National Health Insurance Act, amended in December 2000, expanded the scope of employee medical insurance to include workplaces with one or more employees. As the Enforcement Decree took effect the following year, all employees were subject to employee medical insurance subscription. It was significant in that medical insurance was expanded to all workplaces with one or more employees in the 24 years since the application began in July 1977 for workplaces with 500 or more employees.

In December 1980, the "Act on Special Measures for Rural Health and Medical Care"100) was enacted, providing an advantageous ground for local medical insurance to be implemented nationwide in the 1980s. In consideration of the income level of residents and the distribution of medical facilities, it was stipulated that the residents of the areas determined by the Presidential Decree are eligible to be insured, with the nature of regional health insurance being changed from a voluntary system to a compulsory system. In addition, the coverage of regional medical insurance was based on the administrative unit (si/gun/gu), and cooperative by occupation or job were not restricted by region. Such legal measures by the government greatly helped to prepare the legal and administrative basis for local medical insurance to be implemented.

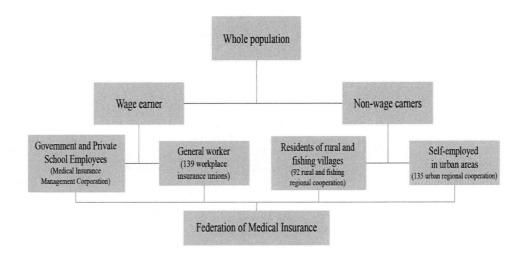

〈Figure 5〉 Medical insurance system (July 1977 – November 1998)

※ Source: Keynote 2017, 40 Years of Health Insurance, and the Road to Becoming a Global Leader – Korea' s Health Insurance Yesterday, Today and Tomorrow

2. Integration into the National Health Insurance System

A. Beginning and Progress of the Debate for Institutional Integration

The Medical Insurance Act, based on legislation passed in December 1963, went into effect on July 1, 1977, to provide medical insurance for employees in workplaces with 500 or more employees. This was managed and operated through 486 medical insurance cooperatives, and the number of medical insurance associations that managed them continued to increase during the process of expanding the covered workplaces. As a result, inefficiencies in management and operation (poor management of cooperatives, financial instability of small cooperatives, etc.) began to emerge. Since the economic feasibility of management was ensured only when the size of the cooperative was certain, small cooperatives were integrated and consolidated.

The political community was in favor of integration, believing that it was a way to realize the national health insurance system. The ruling party (Democratic Party) could not turn away from the aspirations of the majority of the people, who were not eligible for medical insurance benefits, as insurance benefits were only given to some large corporations.

However, many national research institutes as well as the academic community argued that integration was required for national health insurance, but it was difficult to achieve in reality.

Until this time, the debate did not focus on whether to choose integration or cooperatives but on which method would be useful for the early achievement of national health insurance from a practical level rather than an ideological approach.

B. Integration of National Health Insurance

The first debate on the integration of medical insurance took place during the process of integration and consolidation of employee medical insurance cooperatives from 1980 to 1983, and the second debate took place in 1988, when the scope of coverage was expanded to rural areas. After two rounds of debate on integration, the medical insurance operation was maintained to be operated by the cooperative method.

In March 1998, the "Medical Insurance Integration Promotion Group" was launched as an advisory body to the Minister of Health and Welfare to design an integrated system. The Ministry of Health and Welfare prepared the bill for the National Health Insurance Act based on the report of the Medical Insurance Integration Promotion Group and presented it to the National Assembly in December 1998. This bill was intended to consolidate the medical insurance organizations into a single insurer to increase the efficiency of management and operation and the equity of insurance premiums, and to provide comprehensive medical services, including prevention and health promotion, in addition to disease treatment.

The Bill Review Subcommittee under the Health and Welfare Committee of the National Assembly prepared the Bill for the National Health Insurance Act. The key content of the bill was that the National Health Insurance Management Corporation would become the National Health Insurance Corporation and absorb and merge the employee medical insurance cooperatives. After many twists and turns, this bill was enacted and promulgated as the National Health Insurance Act in February 1999.

Based on this Act, the National Health Insurance Service was established in July 2000 by integrating the National Health Insurance Management Corporation and the employee medical insurance cooperatives.

The health insurance integration was actually decided at the end of 1997, and in 1998, it was necessary to decide how to operate the integrated health insurance system. For this, in March 1998, the "Medical Insurance Integration Promotion Group" was launched as an advisory body to the Minister of Health and Welfare. The promotion group carried out work to prepare a bill for an integrated medical insurance system. As a result, in December 1998, a report titled "Measures for the Integration of the Medical Insurance System: Preparation for the Second Leap" was published. It was decided to change the Medical Insurance Review Committee within the Ministry of Health and Welfare to the Health Insurance Review and Coordination Committee and strengthen its functions. The government established the Health Insurance Review and Coordination Committee, which was composed of insurers, health care providers, and representatives of the government and public interest. In 2002, when the "National Health Insurance Financial Consolidation Special Act" was enacted, the name of the committee was changed to the Health Insurance Policy Deliberative Committee.

The organization of the National Medical Insurance Corporation was streamlined to the central and regional offices, and six of the regional offices in Seoul, Busan, Daegu, Incheon, Gwangju, and Daejeon were designated as representative regional offices.

Under the administration led by President Kim Dae−jung, medical insurance integration was promoted with strong momentum, and it was difficult to reverse it any more back to the cooperative method. Nevertheless, opposition was not strong in the process of promoting integration. For this reason, the employee medical insurance cooperatives and the regional medical insurance service were organizationally integrated, but the finances were still divided between the employee medical insurance program and the regional medical insurance program. Although the administration led by President Kim Dae−jung actively promoted financial integration to achieve complete integration, such an effort did not bear fruit. The original plan to integrate the finances of the employee and regional medical insurance programs by January 2002 was delayed by one year and six months to achieve financial integration by July 2003.

3. Expansion of the National Health Insurance System and the Problem of Coverage

With the achievement of National Medical Insurance in 1989, health insurance in Korea was almost completed in terms of its coverage of the entire population. However, the number of pay days and pay items were limited, and even for pay items, the copayment rate was set very high, around 50%. Such a low pay level reduced the financial burden during the introduction of the health insurance system and facilitated the establishment of the system. However, access to medical care was highly dependent on the ability of each household to afford it, and the low−income class had to bear the burden of excessive medical expenses.

Awareness of these issues, along with sustained economic growth, has been the driving force behind a series of steps towards expanding the depth and height of health insurance coverage. Until 2000, the main reforms were the removal of the limit on the number of pay days, the expansion of the scope of pay and the reduction of the copayment rate.

Although the National Health Insurance was achieved in 1989, there was still a limit of 180 pay days combined per year. This limit was maintained until 1993. In other words, services provided beyond 180 days were to be paid in full by the patients themselves. However, by additionally acknowledging various exceptions, insurance benefits were actually expanded.

As demands for reform were constantly raised, in 1994, the limit on the number of pay days was extended to 210 days for the elderly aged 65 and older. In 1995, the limit on the number of pay days was increased to 210 days for all subscribers, and in 2001, the limit on the number of pay days was removed for all subscribers as it was increased to 365 days.

The expansion of insurance benefit items was steadily promoted throughout the entire process of introducing and expanding medical insurance. In the same context, medical insurance was applied to oriental medicine in 1987 and pharmacy in 1989. In the 1990s, the scope of insurance benefits continued to expand as new medical technologies, new drugs, and new materials for treatment continued to be developed with an increase in the public demand for them. In 1992, bone marrow transplantation for those under 40 was included as a medical insurance benefit item, followed by the inclusion of laparoscopic surgery and intraocular lens for cataract surgery in 1993, endoscopic microdiscectomy in 1995, and CT in 1996. In 1997, assisting devices for people with disabilities were included as benefit items, and up to 80% of the purchase cost was supported within the upper limit set by the insurance. Between 1997 and 1999, about 100 items were included as insurance benefit items, such as "single – photon emission computed tomography (SPECT)", "autogenous stem cell transplantation", "percutaneous endovascular stenting", and the "processing cost for using the picture archiving and communication system (PACS)." In 1998, wheelchairs, crutches and canes for the blind were included in the insurance benefits for people with disabilities. From 1999, the drug management fee and the "comprehensive clinical pathology examination fee" were newly introduced. In 2000, health screenings were provided to subscribers and their dependents aged 40 or older, and prenatal examinations were included in the scope of benefits. In 2002, the chronic disease management fee was newly introduced. In 2004, gamma knife surgery was included as an insurance benefit item. In 2005, MRIs, vagus nerve stimulators, and cochlear implants were covered. In 2006, organ transplant surgery was covered, and meals for inpatients were included as insurance benefit items. Furthermore, insurance coverage was gradually expanded for expensive services with high social demands, such as MRI (2010) and ultrasound (2013), starting with serious diseases such as cancers and cardiovascular diseases. The support for assisting devices for people with disabilities (2010) was also expanded, and the support for pregnancy and childbirth treatment expenses (2012) was increased from KRW 200,000 to KRW 500,000 (KRW 700,000 for multiple birth). The insurance started covering oriental physical therapy (2009) in the field of oriental medicine, dental fillings (2009), dentures for the elderly (2012), and tartar removal (2013) in the field of dentistry.

The policy to lower the copayment rate has been actively carried out since the 2000s. In 2000, the target for copayment rate reduction was expanded from those aged 70 or older to those aged 65 or older. In 2001, the outpatient copayment rate for rare and intractable diseases such as cancer and Parkinson's disease was reduced to 20%, and measures to reduce outpatient expenses for cancer patients and 62 rare diseases were applied. In 2005, the out−of−pocket burden for childbirth was eliminated, the outpatient copayment for mental illness was lowered to 20%, and the statutory copayment rate for severe diseases such as cancer was reduced from 20% to 10%. In 2006, copayments for hospitalized children under six years of age were exempted, and the copayment rate for certain cancer screenings was reduced. Those subject to free screenings for the five major cancers (cervical cancer, stomach cancer, breast cancer, colorectal cancer, liver cancer) were expanded to the bottom 50% in terms of the amount of insurance premiums. In 2008, the copayment for hospitalized children under the age of six was raised to 10%. In 2009, the outpatient copayment for tertiary hospital care was increased from 55% to 60% in order to manage demand in line with the health care delivery system. From 2009 to 2010, the copayment for cancer and cardiovascular diseases was further reduced from 10% to 5%, and severe burns (5% copayment) and tuberculosis (10%) were added as diseases subject to assessment exception.

In 2004, the government implemented an "upper limit on copayment" by returning the excess amount above a certain amount for a certain period to the patient.

From 1977, when health insurance was introduced, to 1990, right after national health insurance was achieved, was a period when the focus was on expanding the covered population. As a result, the share of public funds in medical expenses rose sharply. The reason for the double−digit increase in public funds in the 1990s was the expansion of the number of pay days and insurance benefit services. In the 2000s, the increase in the proportion of public finances entered a stagnant state, with the exception of a brief, rapid increase in 2001 in the aftermath of the separation of prescribing and dispensing. In the early 2000s, there was a modest increase in government finances due to the financial crisis in health insurance and measures to strengthen health insurance coverage. In the 2010s, it turned into a decreasing trend (Jeong Hyung−sun, 2015)[33].

---

33) Jeong Hyung−sun (2015), Performance and Tasks of Policies to Strengthen Health Insurance Coverage, HIRA Research Institute, Health Insurance Review and Assessment Service, 2015.

Section 5
Changes in Drugs and the Pharmaceutical Industry

1. Beginning of the Pharmaceutical Industry

Drugs are the most commonly used means of treating diseases and are a health care resource with relatively high accessibility compared to health care workers and other services. They are essential goods, required for many treatments.

Since drugs are substances that are directly administered and affect the human body, the management of their suitability and safety is much more important than for other products. Therefore, the government should prepare regulations on research, production, sales, and quality control in all processes to ensure the provision of safe and effective drugs to consumers.

Drugs also have industrial value as an accumulation of life science and technology and as a result of manufacturing. The pharmaceutical industry is a representative knowledge—based industry, and the continuous development of new drugs is expanding the range of treatable diseases.

A. Inflow of Western Medicine through Open Doors

The Joseon government, which began to accept the modern medical system, put great effort into establishing and implementing the oriental medicine policy as well as establishing the expert standards for drugs, not only by defining the apothecary for the first time but also by introducing licensing regulations. However, after entering colonial rule, Korean wholesalers and retailers of drugs received their supplies from large Japanese wholesalers and sold them to small—scale drug retailers or downsized their business. As the Japanese pharmacists took control of the Korean pharmaceutical industry, the Korean pharmacists also tried to represent their interests. Established in 1908, the Pharmaceutical Industry Association started as a gathering of pharmacists who worked as apothecaries and herbalists. The Pharmaceutical Industry Association, the predecessor of the Korea Oriental Drug Association, was an organization run by Koreans for Koreans in Korea, which was formed in the midst of the pharmacist system, dominated by the Japanese.

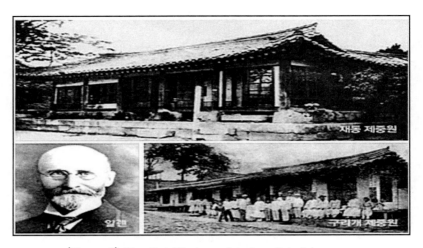

〈Figure 6〉 The first Western-style hospital, Jejungwon.

B. Beginning of the Pharmacy Industry

By the time colonial rule had just begun in 1910, there were virtually no national laws for medicine. This meant that anyone could handle drugs without any restrictions. In 1912, the Japanese Government－General of Korea promulgated the Pharmaceutical Grade Drug Business Control Ordinance and Enforcement Regulations, as well as the regulations for the control of the import and export of narcotics at a level equivalent to the level of regulation by the modern Pharmaceutical Affairs Act.

The establishment of Joseon Pharmacy Academy in 1915 is regarded as the starting point of modern pharmaceutical education. As the academy was found to be effective, the pharmacists felt the limitations of the temporary academy. It was disbanded in 1918 and Joseon Pharmacy School was opened the following year with a two－year program. Joseon Pharmacy School was promoted to Gyeongseong College of Pharmacy in 1930. In 1945, right after liberation, it was reorganized into Seoul College of Pharmacy and re－launched as Seoul National University College of Pharmacy in 1950. In addition, as the number of Korean pharmacists graduated from Joseon Pharmacy School exceeded 100 and the number of licensed pharmacists exceeded 30, the need for a gathering only for Koreans arose. In 1928, the Goryeo Pharmaceutical Association was officially established, and the name was changed to the Korean Pharmaceutical Association in 1948.

C. Appearance of Early Pharmaceutical Industry

With the invasion of sovereignty, the Japanese gained a very advantageous position, owing to the protection of the Governor－General. The economy in Joseon was dominated by Japan, and the market was saturated with Japanese goods. The pharmaceutical industry was no exception, and Japanese pharmacists enjoyed their monopoly status by dominating the import and distribution of Western medicines.

In 1897, Min Byeong—ho and his eldest son Min Kang opened Dongwha Pharmacy. Afterwards, Dongwha Pharmacy officially took the form of a pharmaceutical manufacturer and obtained a license under the 1912 Pharmaceutical Grade Drug Business Revocation Ordinance. Even before that, it showed the quality like a modern enterprise by producing 98 items with permission. In particular, the sale of Insohwan, a digestive tract agent produced by mixing traditional herbal medicines with Western medicines such as alcohol and chloroform obtained from Chejungwon in 1987, has been recognized as the beginning of the Korean pharmaceutical industry. Hwalmyeongsu, a representative product of Dongwha Pharmacy, was first manufactured in 1987. Hwalmyeongsu was Korea's first novel drug, and its trademark and product were registered with the Patent Office of the Japanese Government—General of Korea in 1910. The opening of Dongwha Pharmacy not only marked the beginning of the modern pharmaceutical industry in Korea, but also was a pioneering act in the history of the industry. In 1925, New Il—han temporarily returned to Korea at the invitation of Avison and Underwood. The following year, he founded Yuhan Corporation and started importing drugs from American pharmaceutical companies and supplying them to hospitals. Yuhan Corporation was a Western—style pharmaceutical company that was first introduced to Korea. Kumkang Pharmaceutical was the first pharmaceutical company to succeed in synthesizing drugs using raw materials. Kumkang Pharmaceutical synthesized Salvarson, the first synthetic drug in Korea, to treat syphilis and released it under the name Genvarsan. In addition to this, it also introduced them, Mercurochrome, a disinfectant and Sulfanilamide, a treatment for purulent diseases.

2. Liberation and the Korean War (1945-1953)

A. Shrunk Pharmacy Industry after Liberation

As World War II broke out and heated up, material control for the war system was enforced, and there was a setback in the import of raw materials. The Government—General operated the economy centered on the military industry, and pharmaceutical companies were no exception. Many pharmaceutical companies were consolidated into larger ones, and many pharmacies went out of business. When Japan was defeated and Korea was liberated, the Japanese, who had controlled the domestic pharmaceutical industry, returned to Japan. The domestic industry, which could not overcome the burden of such an absence, shrank sharply.

In a time when medical personnel and facilities were in absolute scarcity right after liberation, medicine contributed greatly to the promotion of public health as a resource with relatively high accessibility. However, the drugs supplied at that time were all very basic nutritional supplements and antibiotics, and there was no choice but to depend on imports. Under the control of the US Military Government, various new drugs, such as penicillin and streptomycin, were introduced into Korea as relief medicines. These drugs captivated the public in an instant, outperforming the existing Western medicines manufactured in Japan at the time.

After liberation, the pharmaceutical industry felt the need for an institution to represent the common interests. Accordingly, the officials founded the Joseon Pharmaceutical Industry Association in 1945, which later became the Korea Pharmaceutical Association.

B. Drifting Pharmaceutical Industry

Even after the establishment of the Korean government, the basics of pharmaceutical administration were still dependent on the military government and the standards of Japanese colonial rule.

The Joseon Pharmaceutical Association, which was established during the Japanese occupation, was an academic organization led by Japanese pharmacists. After liberation, Korean pharmacists formed the Joseon Pharmaceutical Association under the same name in 1946 and continued their research activities. However, with the outbreak of the Korean War, all activities had to be stopped, with key executives of the association being abducted or defecting to North Korea. Afterwards, the inaugural general meeting was held in Busan in 1951, and the name of the association was changed from the Joseon Pharmaceutical Association to the Korean Pharmaceutical Association.

As a result of analysis by the US Economic Cooperation Administration (ECA), it was reported that more than 70% of the pharmaceutical and chemical industries were completely destroyed by the Korean War. During the war, medicine and sanitary materials were absolutely dependent on US aid, but for some items, supplies provided by private companies were also used. Many pharmaceutical companies survived by manufacturing and selling medicines and sanitary products such as analgesics, hemostatic agents, and anthelmintics. The number of casualties and poor evacuation site conditions were also one of the reasons for the rise in pharmaceutical demand.

However, with the entire Korean Peninsula in ruins, there was no sufficient base for the pharmaceutical industry to grow on. Many pharmaceutical factories had to close their doors as there was no way to procure raw materials and subsidiary materials. Until the mid−1950s, the domestic pharmaceutical industry had absolutely no choice but to depend on imports, which led to the heyday of imports of finished products and trade.

3. Efforts to Rebuild the Pharmaceutical Industry

A. Laying the Foundation for Domestic Production

In 1953, the Pharmaceutical Affairs Act was enacted, which established the pharmacist system and the pharmaceutical administration. This meant that the pharmaceutical manufacturing sector was subject to new regulations and supervision. Medicines had to be registered or approved by a managing pharmacist, and the elevated status of pharmacists, the expansion of the profession, and the responsibilities were clearly stipulated.

Until the mid−1950s, the pharmaceutical industry met domestic demand by importing finished products using aid funds from the US International Cooperation Administration (ICA).

As imported drugs flowed in large numbers, the government tried to promote a policy aimed at the substitution of foreign products with domestic product. The plan was to use aid funds to grow pharmaceutical infrastructure and develop similar products while taking the time for imports into the country to settle down. In 1956, the government also promoted the self−production of pharmaceuticals by prohibiting the importation of pharmaceuticals that could be promoted domestically. This policy of the government took into account the insufficient foreign exchange situation and was also implemented with the purpose of fostering domestic companies. However, at that time, the pharmaceutical industry concentrated on the production of finished products that combined them rather than the production of raw materials, and even this involved a very low level of technology, such as launching similar products and competing. However, this enabled the pharmaceutical industry to occupy a firm position as an import substitution industry before the first five−year economic development plan. Although unintentional, it has been a factor in compelling pharmaceutical companies to supply directly to retailers rather than supply competitively through wholesalers.

B. Infrastructure Establishment and System Maintenance

From 1953, the US started to provide aid funds of KRW 200 to 300 million annually. The resumption of production and supply of drugs in the pharmaceutical industry was also owing to the aid. Companies that were allocated funds from the US ICA were not afraid of investment, such as introducing the latest machinery and equipment, which could be considered over−investment, and used the aid funds generously to import raw materials. Representative pharmaceutical companies that received ICA aid until 1961 were able to significantly expand their presence by introducing the latest facilities that could not be found in Korea, such as antibiotics, dehumidification, drying, and aseptic facilities. The revived pharmaceutical industry quickly healed the wounds of war and spurred production activities.

The continued ban on imports of finished drugs by the government under the pretext of protecting the domestic pharmaceutical industry threatened the position of wholesalers. Accordingly, the distribution industry was forced to gradually reduce the proportion of imported goods with a large margin of profit and to deal more domestic goods. In addition, the increase in domestic production increased the contact between producers and intermediaries, and direct sales became a trend. As wholesalers were pushed into a crisis like this, some of them tried to change their industries, and the most representative move the wholesalers made was to enter the pharmaceutical industry.

4. Revival and Development of the Pharmaceutical Industry

A. Establishment of the Pharmaceutical Industry

The government promoted a strong policy to replace imported items with domestic products to encourage the development of the domestic pharmaceutical industry. As a result, imports of finished products began to show a downward curve towards the end of 1950, laying the groundwork for exports. Exports, which have gained momentum, surpassed USD 1 million in 1960. However, there was insufficient regulation on manufacturing, distribution, and pricing, which should have been implemented along with the growth of the industry.

In the 1960s, pharmaceutical companies started to release complex multi−vitamin products. Pharmaceutical companies also started to develop nourishing and tonic agents by adding other drugs to vitamins, and the first product as such was Bacchus by Dong−A Pharmaceutical.

In the 1960s, there was a pressing need to supplement the Pharmaceutical Affairs Ac. In response, the government promulgated the amended Pharmaceutical Affairs Act in 1963. It stipulated the establishment of a pharmacist review committee, the separation of wholesale and retail sales, the prohibition of business in a combined form, and the prohibition of lending licenses. The Pharmaceutical Affairs Act was then amended once more in 1965 to classify medicines into state−approved medicines and addictive and habitual medicines. The separation of wholesale and retail sales and the prohibition of business in a combined form was changed to a sales order, and mandatory provisions for license registration and renewal were newly established. The government also promulgated the facility standard ordinance for the manufacturing, import/export, and sales of pharmacies and pharmaceuticals in 1965 for effective management of pharmaceuticals and tried to raise facility standards by defining manufacturing facilities in detail.

B. Development of the Pharmaceutical Industry

The pharmaceutical industry had been developing as an import substitution industry before the First Five−Year Economic Development Plan in 1962. In the mid−1960s, the upward trend was stagnant due to problems such as the methadone incident and the antibiotic crisis. In the late 1960s, high growth was achieved again as regulations and maintenance were strengthened.

It was difficult to self−produce raw materials at the level of domestic pharmaceutical enterprises in the 1960s. Accordingly, pharmaceutical companies came up with the idea that a joint venture or technology alliance with a foreign company could be an effective import substitution strategy. One of the motivations was that ICA aid could be used for the import of drug substances. The high public preference for foreign trademarks was also a major factor. The first button of this joint venture was made by Handok Pharmaceuticals. Then, JoongAng Pharm, Hanil Pharm, and Yuhan Corporation entered into technical alliances or established joint ventures[34].

---

34) Korea Pharmaceutical and Bio−Pharma Manufacturers Association. "The History of KPMA's 60 Years". 2005.

C. The Golden Age of the Pharmaceutical Industry

In the 1970s, the oil crisis and the resulting economic recession swept the world. However, via export promotion, the government found a breakthrough to achieve substantial growth on its own. The pharmaceutical industry also recorded a rapid growth rate until the mid−1970s, and it was actively used as an opportunity to invest in new businesses or strengthen the internal stability of the company. In addition, the technology alliance that started in the 1960s allowed new product development to flourish in the 1970s. Export promotion and import liberalization, which are national tasks, also encouraged pharmaceutical companies to make improvements. The expansion of health insurance also raised expectations that it would lead to a huge increase in future drug demand. In the 1970s, production of raw materials increased, leading to significant progress in domestic production. In the 1970s, when the proportion of light industry was high, the pharmaceutical industry solidly laid the foundation for novel drug development and firmly established itself as a core industry in Korea.

In 1977, health insurance was launched for businesses with 500 or more employees. The government also designated about 3,000 drugs as insurance drugs prior to implementing health insurance and set the insurance drug prices. Accordingly, in 1976, a cost survey was conducted on 271 pharmaceutical producers, and the price derived in this way was lower than the wholesale price, and the pharmaceutical industry suggested that it was reasonable to add a certain percentage to the average price. In addition, it was difficult to investigate using the ex−officio due diligence system, and there was no difference between the calculated factory shipment price and the shipment price reported by pharmaceutical companies. Therefore, the notification system reported by companies through the association has been converted to a reimbursement system since 1982.

In the 1970s, the Ministry of Health and Social Affairs implemented a drug substance protection system that prohibited imports of drug substances that could be produced domestically unless they were more expensive than the international market price. This was intended to promote the development of domestic technology and cultivate international competitiveness. The Ministry of Health and Social Affairs also introduced a policy to protect the approval for up to five years for the first drug substance developed in Korea. As the pharmaceutical industry grew, a drug management system was introduced to facilitate the supply of outstanding products. The government introduced Korea Good Manufacturing Practice (KGMP) in 1977 to minimize defective products in the manufacturing stage. This meant that all manufacturing processes, from raw materials to finished products, were meticulously managed in order to reduce the production of any defective products caused by worker negligence. In reality, the government judged that it would be difficult to complete facility investments in accordance with KGMP in a short period of time and recommended voluntary implementation to pharmaceutical companies. The first KGMP certified company appeared in 1985.

D. Continuation of the High-growth Trend

As a result of the establishment of the college of pharmacy at universities across the country in the 1950s and 1960s, the number of registered pharmacists increased rapidly in the 1970s. In the 10 years from 1970 to 1979, about 10,000 new pharmacists were produced. This led to side effects such as a surge in the number of new pharmacies and excessive competition. As such, the oversupply of pharmacists was raised as a problem, and the Korean Pharmaceutical Association focused on reducing the quota of the college of pharmacy while expanding the work scope of pharmacists. However, it was difficult to expect the university authorities to reduce the quota on their own.

With the development of the pharmaceutical industry, the demand for pharmacists in production and distribution management has increased rapidly. It was not at a sufficient level, but it helped with addressing the issue of expanding the work scope of pharmacists to some extent.

Despite the 1973 oil crisis, the pharmaceutical industry achieved remarkable growth. The production of pharmaceuticals, which was less than KRW 50 billion in 1971, increased to KRW 658.5 billion in 1980. Exports also reached more than $70 million at the end of the 1970s, up from $3.5 million at the end of the 1960s[35].

However, there were some limitations. Infrastructure construction or technology investment fell behind to make way for securing pharmaceutical facilities and raw materials. Pharmaceutical companies realized the need for facility expansion in the mid−1970s. However, expansion was difficult due to the lack of funds and measures preventing new construction or expansion in several factories.

The rapid growth of the pharmaceutical industry, overproduction, and oversupply put the wholesale industry into a crisis. This became fully apparent in the 1970s, when pharmaceutical companies increased the volume of direct sales to drug retailers. In addition, large pharmacies began to open, and intermediary wholesalers appeared. Brokers also started to appear, handling drugs without any permission. As the proportion of brokers increased, the distribution order became blurry. They also evaded taxes through unusual sales practices. This activity of brokers weakened the pharmaceutical wholesale industry and led to the bankruptcy of wholesalers that followed in the early 1970s. In addition, the reduced supply of oil due to the oil crisis led to limited production of pharmaceuticals and took a toll on the pharmaceutical industry as a whole.

In 1977, the value added tax (VAT) system was introduced. This has had a huge impact on all trades in the pharmaceutical industry. From business policy to pharmacy management, all areas were affected, and it became an opportunity for changes in drug distribution. The increased amount of tax payment hindered the pharmaceutical industry's ability to secure cash, leading to double hardship and financial difficulties. The relatively slow fund rotation caused cash pressure. The introduction of VAT affected the price the most. Although a price increase was inevitable, the government advised against raising retail prices. This led to the observation that everyone in the pharmaceutical industry would have to accept sales without margins. However, the

---

35) Korea Pharmaceutical and Bio−Pharma Manufacturers Association. "The History of KPMA's 60 Years" 2005.

introduction of the VAT system promoted the disclosure of tax data, which had been hidden in the pharmaceutical industry, and served as an opportunity to clean up the absurdity in the transaction process.

5. Opening of the Pharmaceutical Industry through Globalization

A. Transition to the Relaxation Period

In the 1980s, with the introduction of the national health insurance system, all citizens were able to receive medical benefits. Although the pharmaceutical industry continued to grow steadily and surpassed KRW 1 trillion in production, it did not show the same growth rate as in the 1970s. Raw material prices in Japan and Europe, which were highly dependent on imports, soared due to the strong dollar maintained in the 1980s. Under cost–cutting conditions, the domestic pharmaceutical industry had to work extra hard to stay afloat.

There were several cases of high–level drug substance development, such as cephalosporin integration by Hanmi Pharm. However, the self–sufficiency of raw materials in the domestic pharmaceutical industry, which had risen sharply until the 1970s, began to decline. Accordingly, the necessity for domestic production of drug substances was highlighted once again, but in the harsh reality, the pharmaceutical industry had no choice but to rely on technology transfer from foreign companies, and due to the limits, that could not be supplemented by its own efforts.

In the 1980s, the government presented a plan to promote technological innovation and internationalization, and to promote the opening of all fields. In 1983, the Ministry of Health and Social Affairs announced that it would allow the import of specific drug substances and finished drugs as a first step. It was an opening policy based on efforts to reduce the side effects as much as possible by allowing the import of items that were not mainly produced domestically and had international competitiveness. After that, by 1987, import liberalization expanded to almost all items of drug substances and finished products.

In 1981, the government raised the minimum foreign investment limit to more than $100,000 and the maximum investment rate to 100%. As a result, multinational pharmaceutical companies began to approach for joint ventures based on the domestic market's growth potential. Although there were many positive aspects to the entry of multinational companies into Korea, it was not without negative aspects either. Domestic companies expected that the joint venture would contribute to the development of the industry through advanced technology and management techniques, but the joint ventures mainly focused on the production of finished products and an increase in sales. There were also many ventures that did not comply with the conditions for domestic raw material production.

The government introduced the standard retail price system for all pharmaceuticals in 1984. This system was introduced to correct overrepresentation of drug prices and disorderly distribution, which was implemented in the form of a sticker indicating the drug price at the final distribution stage.

B. Efforts to the Market Opening

The basic work of the GMP system started in the 1970s, and it was enacted and announced in 1984. After that, three companies, Yuhan Corporation, Dong−A Pharm, and Bukwang Pharm, were designated as KGMP−certified companies in 1985 through assessment. This meant that Korea's pharmaceutical manufacturing and management capabilities had reached an international level. KGMP certification was a project that required a lot of funds, but the introduction of the system was a trend of the times, and a consensus was formed that business expansion would be difficult without a base for producing high quality drugs. Since 1994, KGMP certification has been made mandatory for all drug manufacturers[36].

The introduction of a substance patent means that even if a pharmaceutical company holds a patent on an improved method, the technology can only be used after obtaining the permission of the patent holder who first developed the substance; that is, the technology is subject to subordination. In 1985, a delegation from the International Pharmaceutical Patent Association visited Korea and pressured the adoption of the substance patent system. Since 1987, the material patent system has been fully implemented[37]. As a result, the pharmaceutical industry was faced with the task of building independent R&D capabilities and international competitiveness. Pipeline products also put a big brake on the domestic pharmaceutical industry. It was a policy to restrict the approval of domestic analogues for products that had obtained US patents after January 1980 and were not sold in the US and Korea before 1987. It was a policy that guaranteed patent rights even after the protection period for material patents, and the domestic pharmaceutical industry had to bear the blow.

Among these policies, domestic pharmaceutical companies have begun to turn their attention to the importance of R&D for new drug. As a result, nine pharmaceutical companies started developing new drugs in earnest, and in the early 1990s, progress was made to the point where they completed animal testing and entered clinical trials. In addition, with the introduction of substance patents, multinational pharmaceutical companies decided that it was more advantageous to establish a joint venture through direct investment rather than a technology alliance. The establishment of Korea Good Laboratory Practice (KGLP), Korea Good Clinical Practice (KGCP), and Korea Good Supplying Practice (KGSP), following KGMP, reflected such a decision. Since the introduction of the substance patent system, vigorous research on natural products has been conducted, creating a boom in herbal medicines. Pharmaceutical companies took an interest in Oriental medicine as it was not only easy to secure natural resources, but also relatively free from the influence of advanced countries.

On July 1, 1989, the era of national health insurance application for the entire nation began as the urban poor and the self−employed were added to the beneficiaries of insurance. The participation of pharmacies in health insurance was also a part of the project. Although the pharmaceutical association had always insisted on the early implementation of the separation of prescribing and dispensing, the

---

36) Ministry of Health and Social Affairs. "Health and Social Affairs White Paper". 1990; Ministry of Health and Welfare. "Health and Welfare White Paper". 1995.

37) Lim Geun−young. A Study on Efficient IPR Trade Policy Directions. Korea Institute of Intellectual Property. 2006.

government designated pharmacies as health care institutions in July 1989 and notified them to implement a partial separation of prescribing and dispensing within the insurance program. As a result, the members of the pharmaceutical association closed their establishments and condemned the government. In the end, the Ministry of Health and Social Welfare, which compromised with the Pharmaceutical Association, redefined insurance benefits by implementing a three−stage co−payment system for patients, limiting the number of doses administered, and limiting the drugs covered. On October 1, 1989, insurance benefits started being applied to pharmacies as well.

C. Heightened Sense of Crisis following Structural Change

In the domestic pharmaceutical industry, which was completely open due to the market opening measures in the 1980s, structural changes and trials were expected. It had to develop self−reliance by adapting to the rules of the globalization era, moving away from a state of complacency in the domestic market. In addition, it was an era in which the environment was changing, such as health care coverage for the entire nation, the upcoming separation of prescribing and dispensing, the reinforcement of intellectual property rights protection, and the increasing market pressure on developing countries. In order to overcome the difficult reality of introducing technology, the domestic pharmaceutical industry has devised an attempt to strengthen marketing and R&D capabilities through strategic alliances as well as mergers and acquisitions. There was a movement to strengthen investment in research to supplement new products and to lay the foundation for novel drug development. Nevertheless, companies could not avoid the effects of aggressive marketing by multinational pharmaceutical companies and the economic downturn, falling into a vicious cycle of low growth and low profits.

The government declared war on drugs in 1991 to directly solve the problem of drug abuse. The following year, an anti−drug campaign centered on the Korean Pharmaceutical Association was launched, adding to the status of pharmacists as experts in medicine and establishing the concept of their service to public health.

In the early 1990s, the domestic pharmaceutical industry began to invest in research with an aggressive attitude to develop new drugs. The government was also aware of the seriousness of the reality of the pharmaceutical industry, and there was a perception that it was impossible to solve the problem without government support. After the government established the basic plan for new drug development in 1990, it started supporting research expenses in 1991. In addition, the Ministry of Science and Technology has supported the development of new drugs since 1992 as a leading technology development project. Other government ministries and agencies also expanded their support to include the pharmaceutical sector in the high−tech development support projects.

As a result, drug technology exports also flourished, resulting in LG's transfer of a USD 15 million cephalosporin material patent to GlasoSmithKline and Hanmi Pharm's transfer of microemulsion formulation technology to Novartis. In addition, UNDP established the International Vaccine Research Institute in 1997 to contribute to the promotion of human welfare through vaccine research and development, and selected Korea as a host country.

D. Preparing for the 21st Century

In 1997, the Korean government requested the IMF for liquidity adjustment funds. The pharmaceutical industry could not escape the crisis. The structure of the pharmaceutical industry has collapsed due to the sharp rise in the exchange rate and manufacturing costs, exchange rate losses, insufficient solvency, and chain bankruptcies of wholesalers. However, the IMF did not simply have negative impacts. This served as an opportunity that once again emphasized the importance of maximizing drug distribution efficiency, large–scale expansion through mergers and acquisitions, as well as integration, avoiding chaos, and making transparent transactions.

Korea joined the OECD in 1996 and revised the drug safety test management standards accordingly in 1998 for international harmonization. Regulations have been relaxed to allow foreign test results to be applied in Korea without having to conduct a phase 3 clinical trial in Korea. As for drugs developed in foreign countries, international participation was facilitated by allowing participation in multinational trials as long as the reliability of the results of non–clinical or clinical trials was ensured at all stages.

In 1998, the market share of prescription drugs surpassed that of over–the–counter drugs, and the same phenomenon occurred the following year, signaling the entry into the era of prescription drugs. On the other hand, the pharmaceutical raw material manufacturing industry was focused on seeking self–rescue measures such as abandoning or reducing production and exporting. Furthermore, the price drop of expensive new drug substances and existing raw materials as a result of substance patents exacerbated the phenomenon. Accordingly, drug substance manufacturers turned their eyes to the production of raw materials for antibiotics and tried to develop overseas markets. However, since export requires bulk good manufacturing practice (BGMP), the introduction of this system caused a huge burden of facility investment.

In the mid–1990s, companies realized the need for thorough monitoring and supervision of drugs and foods, and an organization similar to the US FDA was required for this. The Korea Centers for Food and Drug Safety, launched in 1996, took over the functions of food and drug approval and monitoring from the Ministry of Health and Welfare, the functions of food and drug collection and inspection from the National Institutes of Health, and the functions of toxicity and safety research from the Institute for Health and Safety. The Korea Centers for Food and Drug Safety were promoted to the Korea Food and Drug Administration in 1998 and took over most of the functions of the Pharmacopoeia and the Food and Drug Administration.

The 1990s were also a time when numerous efforts were made to increase competitiveness in the global market. This may have boosted domestic pharmaceutical–related patent applications in the 1990s. In the early 1990s, the number of patent applications stood at about 600 per year, but by 1999, it nearly doubled to more than 1,200. The same was true for technology transfers. Starting with the technology transfer of Hanmi Pharm in 1989, Lucky Goldstar, Yuhan Corporation, and Hanmi Pharm achieved technology transfers of more than USD 10 million.

In 1997, the first domestic novel drug Sunpla was developed, and it was approved for commercialization in 1999. Sunpla was a platinum–complex anticancer drug, and it was a product that supplemented the shortcomings of second–generation anticancer drugs. It was not an imitation of a foreign product, but a product developed purely in Korea through all development processes, thus playing a pioneering role in suggesting a novel drug development model for Korea. It was the first achievement in about 10 years since SK started its development in 1990. The news that Sunpla had obtained the approval was a feat that motivated the domestic pharmaceutical industry to develop novel drugs and gave confidence.

E. Era of Separation of Prescribing and Dispensing

The separation of prescribing and dispensing was aimed at protecting public health from misuse and abuse of medicines by correcting wrong practices regarding the use of medicines, reducing the use of unnecessary medicines to reduce national medical expenses, and promoting the patient's right to know and the level of medical service[38]. The revision of the Pharmaceutical Affairs Act, including the enforcement of the separation of prescribing and dispensing in 1999, was decided to come into effect in 2000.

In 2001, the financial difficulties of health insurance emerged as a new problem. It was not an unexpected problem. The problem was rooted in the accumulated deficit since the insurance cooperative days before health insurance integration, which had gradually expanded. Another factor was the fact that the fee was raised by about 50% for one year during the promotion of the separation of prescribing and dispensing[39]. Although the government denied the possibility of the crisis caused by fiscal exhaustion, it gradually came true. Several policies to curb the increase in drug costs were promoted, such as removing the drug price bubble by expanding the actual transaction price survey, paying a certain percentage of the difference in drug prices as an incentive when dispensing loans, and lowering the price of generic drugs From this point on, adequacy evaluations to monitor drug use and provide feedback on the results of antibiotics and expensive drugs with high potential for misuse began to be performed.

Despite the government's efforts, health insurance drug expenditures kept rising sharply. The share of pharmaceuticals in health insurance medical expenses rose from 23.5% in 2001 to 29.2% in 2005. A complete overhaul of the drug pricing method was essential. In response, the Ministry of Health and Welfare announced a plan to optimize drug costs in 2006. The contents included measures such as changing the drug listing method to a positive list, establishing a comprehensive pharmaceutical information center, and adjusting the price of original drugs when producing generic drugs. In order to promote the proper use of drugs and prevent the use of prohibited drugs, a drug prescription dispensing support system was established and installed in the insurance claim programs of all health care institutions in 2008. A legal basis was established by including the obligation of pharmacists to check prescriptions as well as the obligatory response of doctors. For discontinued items due to safety−related reasons, prescription and dispensing decreased by 98.1% and 100%, respectively. Then, in 2010, the Drug Utilization Review (DUR) managed by the Health Insurance Review and Assessment Service was introduced to prevent the use of prohibited drugs or duplicate prescriptions.

---

38) Ministry of Welfare, "70 Years of Health and Welfare" vol.2 Health Care, 2016, p.529

39) Cha Heung−bong. Process of the Separation of Prescribing and Dispensing. Jipmoondang. 2006.

F. Efforts for Advancement

The IMF financial crisis put pharmaceutical companies into a structural transition period. Efforts to rationalize management, such as attracting foreign capital and strategic alliances, as well as reduction through restructuring, were essential. In addition, mergers and acquisitions were carried out in all areas to introduce new products and restore sales power. Fortunately, these efforts came as a result of increased sales as the demand for pharmaceuticals increased in the aftermath of the separation of prescribing and dispensing in the 2000. It was the result of a combination of factors such as reducing debt through continuous restructuring of pharmaceutical companies, reducing financial expenses, stabilizing fixed costs, and reducing manufacturing costs due to stable exchange rates. Fortunately, in 2004, most pharmaceutical companies began to transition to a recovery phase, with their production performance finally exceeding KRW 10 trillion.

In the 21st century, the production technology and facilities of pharmaceutical companies have risen to a considerable level, and companies that only focus on exporting finished products have emerged. Even so, exports to advanced markets in the United States and Europe, excluding Southeast Asia and Japan, were still poor. In addition, many pharmaceutical companies have yet to perceive the export market as only a secondary market to the domestic market. The trade imbalance problem has also been exacerbated, mainly due to the aging population and high−tech new drugs. Pharmaceutical companies are investing huge amounts of money to build current good manufacturing practice (cGMP) factories to produce products meeting the standards in the US and Europe.

GLP was established as new drugs were actively developed, Investigational New Drug (IND) was established in 2002 for clinical trial plans, and Institutional Review Board (IRB) were introduced in 2007 in order to facilitate clinical trials.

In 2010, the Ministry of Health, Welfare and Family Affairs announced a market price reimbursement system as part of a plan to make drug transaction and drug price systems transparent. It was a system reflecting the opinion that improvement was inevitable, as the existing system evoked a trade practice called "rebates." The main purpose of the market price reimbursement system is to pay a portion of the difference as an incentive when a health care institution purchases a drug at a lower price than the advertised price and lowers the drug price the following year. The government wanted this to cut drug costs and eradicate illegal rebates. In 2010, the drug rebate dual penalty system was enacted. As a result, health care personnel or workers in medical institutions were subject to imprisonment or fines if they received rebates from pharmaceutical companies. This was a system introduced to improve the inadequacy of the previous one, in which only the giver could be punished, not the receiver who received a rebate. The low−price purchase incentive system was abolished in 2014, and the low−price purchase incentive and usage reduction incentive systems are currently being implemented.

In 2012, the Ministry of Health and Welfare announced that it would implement drug price reductions for registered drugs. The drug price cut was introduced to reduce insurance premiums for the purpose of stabilizing insurance finances. The pharmaceutical association expressed strong opposition to this, but it was ignored by the government, which ultimately led to a decline in business performance. Although several attempts were made to compensate for the loss in sales, such as diversifying the business or strengthening over—the—counter drugs, they failed to generate sufficient income. The drug price cut also brought changes to sales, as rebates became impossible and the prices of originals and generics became the same, leading to customers preferring originals over generics.

After Sunpla obtained approval from the Food and Drug Administration as the first novel drug in 1999, domestic pharmaceutical companies have continued to develop novel drugs. In particular, LG's antibacterial agent, Factive, was approved by the US FDA in 2003, boasting the world—class level of Korean pharmaceutical technology. This named Korea as one of the world—class new drug development countries along with advanced European countries and the United States. In addition, novel drugs derived from natural products are continuously being developed, which are attracting more attention due to their relatively few adverse effects compared to synthetic drugs and the advantage Korea has in their development due to its long tradition and history of oriental medicine. Celltrion's work in 2012, Remsima, also deserves attention as it is the first biosimilar drug in Korea.

Based on such efforts, the Ministry of Health and Welfare selected innovative pharmaceutical companies in 2012. It was a project prepared for the purpose of nurturing and developing the pharmaceutical industry as a driving force for the future. As an incentive, companies selected as innovative pharmaceutical companies were given priority to participate in national projects, and benefits such as tax support and exemption from research facility charges were also given. In addition, benefits such as investment in public funds and priority loans for policy funds were provided.

6. Policy Direction for the Pharmaceutical Industry

Drugs are one of the most important resources in the Korean health care system, which have made remarkable progress along with the development of the country. The pharmaceutical industry, which depended on imports and supplied only a limited number of medicines immediately after liberation, achieved domestic production through government support and technology introduction and grew significantly along with economic development and the national health insurance system. Koreans now have access to a very diverse spectrum of drugs, from cutting—edge novel drugs to everyday drugs. In addition, the level of production and quality control, such as GMP and GLP, has also been greatly improved.

The drugs produced in Korea, however, are still insufficient to compete on an equal footing with the products from advanced countries in the global market. It will be necessary to carry out more thorough quality control and to be recognized for its quality at home and abroad. The increase in the use of drugs with the development of novel drugs as well as the aging population is starting to become the main cause of the rise in health care costs. This is a phenomenon experienced by most developed countries, and various policies have already been implemented to effectively manage the cost. The cost increase due to the aging population and the increase in chronic diseases is expected to continue in the future. In order to achieve optimal effects with limited resources, continued efforts to seek a balance in expenditures through cost—effective drug use and reasonable pricing will be required.

Now that the aging population and the increase in the prevalence of chronic diseases have become common phenomena, a transition from the conventional acute disease—centered health care system to a lifelong health care system is required. In addition, socially essential medical care should be provided by establishing a safety net through the expansion of medical care for the vulnerable and the establishment of a response system for new infectious diseases. Lastly, investment and support for health care industries such as drugs and medical devices are required. It is necessary to foster and support the global health industry by nurturing the industry to ensure the quality, price, and accessibility of health care services[40].

---

40) Choi Byung—ho et al. "Analysis of major policy issues." Korea Institute for Health and Social Affairs, 2007.

Section 6

Changes in Health Promotion Policies

1. Concretization of Health Promotion Policies and Establishment of Comprehensive Plans

The promotion of public health has been extended beyond passive activities to prevent or remove harmful factors from active and proactive activities to create an environment in which people can live a healthy life and take care of their own health. The duty of the government to prepare an environment for health promotion and provide support was embodied in the "National Health Promotion Act," granting the necessary authority to the government to realize it.

The government established a pan−government mid−to long−term comprehensive plan that provided directions for public health promotion and disease prevention policies based on Article 4 of the National Health Promotion Act by forming a committee with citizens and experts. Since 2002, this plan has been implemented in three phases (phase 1 from 2002 to 2005, phase 2 from 2006 to 2010, and phase 3 from 2011 to 2020) with the goal of extending healthy lifespans and improving health equity.

Meanwhile, the government has established and operated the Korea Health Promotion Institute since 2014 for the efficient operation of the health promotion fund created in accordance with the National Health Promotion Act and the smooth promotion of projects.

2. Community-based Health Promotion Project

Based on the belief that the national health promotion project should be provided in the living environment of the people, the subject of the health promotion project should be the local community. Accordingly, the law provides obligations, powers, and resources for all members of local governments and local communities to participate in this project. The contents of the project included "health education and health counseling, nutrition management, oral health management, screening and prescription for early detection of disease, survey on community health issues, and operation of other health classes." From the pilot implementation stage of the health promotion projects to the present, health promotion projects in Korea seem synonymous with health promotion projects at public health centers. Since this project can be voluntarily carried out in various contexts, the channel for participation is currently open to organizations other than public health centers. The tasks that can be entrusted include "a healthy life support project, health education, survey/research for health promotion and prevention of chronic degenerative diseases, health screening, and physical activity for health promotion."

The health promotion projects of public health centers started in September 1998 with nine health promotion pilot health center projects. As the public health centers carried out the project with a focus on primary and secondary prevention activities at the time, it was difficult to handle the new areas of health promotion. The main contents of the pilot project included hypertension prevention, stroke prevention, school health, and oral health, and from the second half of 1999, health life practice projects such as smoking cessation, exercise, and nutrition, which were differentiated from existing health projects, were partially supplemented. As the project expanded, from October 2002, 100 public health centers across the country were allowed to selectively operate the four health life practice projects of smoking cessation, temperance, and nutrition in consideration of local conditions. It was around this time that the health promotion project came to be understood as a separate project area. Since 2005, health promotion projects have been implemented at public health facilities around the country, with four areas of healthy living practice and a smoking cessation clinic developed.

Since 2008, the "Regional Specialized Health Behavior Improvement" project has been operating to improve health promotion projects at public health centers. In the meantime, the project was conducted with a population group with health risk behaviors based on objective health indicators by promoting subjective targets by region. In order to enhance the effectiveness and efficiency of the project, the self−contained program was expanded and linked to various programs that engage the local community to create a healthy environment and ensure system improvement in a comprehensive way.

The "Integrated Health Promotion Program in the Local Community" was pushed to increase the satisfaction of the public with health center health promotion projects in order to alleviate the challenges faced in promoting health promotion projects at public health facilities. The local government reorganized the budget for each field of health promotion according to local circumstances and provided integrated services for the target.

3. Examples of Health Promotion Projects: Development and Change in Smoking Cessation Policy

A. Reduction of Smoking Rate through Pricing Policy

Representative methods for lowering the smoking rate are divided into non−price policies and price policies. These non−price policies include education, publicity, and non−smoking advertisements; regulation of tobacco company promotions and advertisements; writing of smoking warnings; and restrictions on smoking areas and designating non−smoking areas. In Korea, non−price policies have been mainly implemented. The smoking rate decreased by 9.4% following the price increase for cigarettes was raised by KRW 300 in 2001, and it decreased by 5.5% following the price increase for cigarettes by KRW 500 in 2004.

The cigarette levy is officially known as the "National Health Promotion Tax," which is also known as the tobacco tax, as it has only been levied on cigarettes since 2002. In 1995, when the "National Health Promotion Act" was enacted, a levy was imposed on the tobacco business operators (KRW 2 per pack of cigarettes) and the insurers of health insurance (5% of the health insurance preventive health project cost) in order to secure and support the financial resources necessary for the smooth implementation of the national health promotion project. As it was decided to impose a charge of KRW 150 per 20 cigarettes when the law was amended in 2002, the levy imposed on the insurers has been eliminated. The fund raised from the levy includes health life support projects, health education and data development, survey research for health promotion and prevention of chronic degenerative diseases, screening for early detection of diseases, national nutrition and oral health management, and health promotion projects conducted by public health center directors. Recently, in December 2014, the levy was increased from KRW 354 to KRW 841, with a cigarette price increase of KRW 2,000 per pack. In 2015, the total amount of the National Health Promotion Fund was KRW 2.7189 trillion. Among them, the amount of support for health insurance subscribers was KRW 1.5185 trillion, and the cost of health promotion was KRW 1.2004 trillion.

B. Reduction of Smoking Rates through Non-price Policies

Non−price policies implemented by the government include prohibiting youth from purchasing cigarettes, attaching smoking warnings, and limiting advertisements. However, the most prominent policies are the designation of smoking areas and the imposition of fines for smokers.

In Korea, there are laws and regulations that restrict the sale of cigarettes, such as the National Health Promotion Act, the Youth Protection Act, and the Tobacco Business Act. The sale of cigarettes to youths under the age of 19 is prohibited (Article 26 of the Youth Protection Act), and the sale of cigarettes by mail or electronic transaction (Article 12, Paragraph 3 of the Tobacco Business Act) is also prohibited. In addition, cigarette vending machines can only be installed in places where juveniles cannot access them, and in July 2004, an adult authentication device was attached to the vending machines (Article 9 of the "National Health Promotion Act"). In 1989, smoking warnings were applied to cigarette packaging, and since then, it has been stipulated that warnings about smoking being harmful to health should be displayed on the front and back of cigarette packaging (increased from 20% to 30% since April 2005), stickers or posters affixed to business offices of designated retailers, and magazine advertisements.

The Ministry of Health and Welfare enacted the National Health Promotion Act in 1995, requiring some facilities, such as large buildings, performance halls, academies, large—scale stores, tourist accommodations, wedding ceremonies, indoor gymnasiums, medical institutions, social welfare facilities, and transportation facilities, to have non—smoking areas. The Ministry of Health and Welfare enacted the National Health Promotion Act in 1995, requiring some facilities, such as large buildings, performance halls, academies, large—scale stores, tourist accommodations, wedding ceremonies, indoor gymnasiums, medical institutions, social welfare facilities, and transportation facilities, to have non—smoking areas. In 1999, a bathhouse was newly added, and in 2003, game and PC cafes, large restaurants, comic book cafes, government buildings, and childcare facilities were newly added, while non—smoking areas were also expanded. In 2006, the non—smoking area designated mainly for large—scale offices was expanded to include small offices, factories, and local government offices. The Ministry of Health and Welfare has been reviewing more facilities to designate them as non—smoking areas in the future. In addition, in order to strengthen regulations to the level recommended by the Framework Convention on Tobacco Control (FCTC), laws and systems have been further reinforced in terms of raising cigarette prices, introducing smoking warning pictures, strengthening warning signs, and expanding non—smoking areas.

The government joined the World Health Organization Framework Convention on Tobacco Control in 2005 and is a member of the Conference of Parties (COP). The Conference of the Parties is held every two years. The fifth meeting was held in November 2012 in Seoul, and the "Protocol to Eliminate Illicit Trade in Tobacco Products" and the "Seoul Declaration", which declared the joint response of member countries to the intervention and obstruction of tobacco companies, were adopted as a joint initiative between the Republic of Korea and Uruguay.

4. Promotion of Policies to Improve Nutrition

A. Establishment of Master Plan

At the national level, to solve nutritional problems caused by an increase in income levels, low fertility and aging, nutritional imbalances in which both nutritional deficiency and excess coexist, disparity between income classes, an increase in the obese population and chronic diseases, and an increase in the frequency of eating out and use of processed foods, policies are needed. Based on the reflection that such policies were carried out sporadically and overlappingly, the "First Master Plans for Basic National Nutrition Management (2012 to 2016)" was established (August, 2012)[41].

B. Development of Nutrition Management Program

The nutrition improvement policy aims to promote the improvement of nutrition through the development of relevant competencies in people. Through the computer program operation event for nutrition diagnosis, the experience of reviewing one's eating habits and evaluating the desired dietary habits, such as the amount and calories of food according to one's age and activity, is provided.

In addition, support projects tailored to each life cycle were carried out, which applied to pregnant women (pregnant, child−bearing, and lactating women) and infants up to a certain age (under 6 years old) of households with incomes below the minimum cost of living who are determined to have nutritional risk factors. It was a national nutrition support project that provided nutrition education and specific supplementary foods for proper nutrition over a certain period of time.

C. Establishment of Nutritional Component Database for Each Food

The nutritional component database construction project for each food is a project that aims to secure nutritional component data for commercial foods in order to establish basic data for nutritional status evaluation and policy establishment. Furthermore, it is contributing to revealing the relationship between diet and chronic degenerative diseases by understanding the levels of people's nutrient intake, which has been difficult to determine, and is being utilized in preparing policies to improve desirable eating habits.

D. Korea National Health and Nutrition Examination Survey

The Korea National Health and Nutrition Examination Survey (KNHANES) is conducted for the purpose of producing national representative statistics on the health and nutritional status of Koreans and supporting them to be used in health policy establishment and evaluation. In particular, the information on this project serves as the basis for the calculation of the indicators of the National Health Promotion Plan and is provided as an international health indicator. Above all, it is used for statistical calculation by building an analysis database in the year following the survey.

---

41) Articles 7 and 8 of the "National Nutrition Management Act" enacted in 2010 as the legal basis.

5. Changes in the System for Mental Health Promotion

A. Establishment of Mental Health-related Health Care Institutions

The current "Seoul National Hospital" run by the government was opened as a "National Mental Hospital" in Junggok—dong in 1962, according to the "Medical Facility Restoration Plan" at the end of 1956. In May 2002, it was renamed "Seoul National Hospital."

At the beginning of its establishment, the main purpose of this institution was to provide psychiatric beds, but as mental health policy changed from the management of mentally ill patients to rehabilitation and again to the promotion of mental health for all people, the activities of national psychiatric hospitals established by the government changed.

B. Expansion of Community-based Mental Health Projects

Community mental health projects were attempted in some parts of the 1970s, and since the mid—1980s, the need for deinstitutionalization and rehabilitation of mentally ill people has been raised and has been expanding.

The community mental health project reached a turning point in revitalization with the "Mental Health Act," enacted in 1995. The Mental Health Act gave priority to policy interest and support in establishing an integrated mental health service provision system for early detection; providing counseling, treatment, and rehabilitation services; and promoting the rehabilitation of mentally ill people in the local community. The institution that played a pivotal role above all else in establishing this community—based treatment and rehabilitation system was the mental health center. The mental health center project was first implemented in 1998, and the name was changed to the mental health promotion center in February 2013. As of March 2015, 197 community mental health promotion centers and 13 metropolitan mental health promotion centers were established.

C. Implementation of Policies for Suicide Prevention

In our society, the suicide rate has increased rapidly due to the background of an elderly population increase, economic polarization, and the amplification of social conditions such as the 1997 IMF economic crisis. The suicide rate was 22.6 people in 2003, exceeding 20 people for the first time, peaking at over 30 people from 2009 to 2011, and then reaching a very high level of 26.6 people in 2018.

Suicide is a catastrophic phenomenon that affects individuals and society, and it is necessary to prevent it. In September 2004, the government prepared the "First Comprehensive Plan for Suicide Prevention," which included suicide prevention counseling, culture creation, and programs for mutual support among citizens. Meanwhile, in order to systematically promote suicide prevention projects, the "Act on the Prevention of Suicide and the Creation of Culture of Respect for Life" was enacted in March 2011 and implemented one year later. In accordance with this Act, while aiming to spread awareness of respect for life and prevent suicide in society, projects such as establishing a master plan for suicide prevention every five years, conducting a survey, providing counseling and treatment, and operating a suicide hazard information prevention system.

D. Prevention of Excessive Drinking

Article 8 of the "National Health Promotion Act" enacted in January 1995 (smoking cessation and temperance campaigns, etc.) stipulates that national and local government education and publicity about the health risks of excessive drinking, obligatory labeling of warning phrases on alcoholic beverage containers, and support for surveys and research on temperance. The Youth Protection Act, enacted in March 1997, defined alcohol as a drug harmful to youth and stipulated the prohibition of selling or lending alcohol. However, the burden of drinking in Korean society still exists, and the consequences of domestic violence and drunk driving accidents are serious, calling for measures. In order to prevent this, the Alcohol Counseling Center (2000) was established, and the name was changed to the "Integrated Addiction Management Support Center," which included Internet, gambling, and drug addiction, and the function was reorganized. As of 2015, a total of 50 locations were in operation.

E. Efforts to Improve Awareness of Mental Illness

One of the main purposes of the enactment of the "Mental Health Act" was to protect the human rights of people with mental illness through the sharing and diffusion of correct awareness of mental illness.

In 2001, on the occasion of setting the theme of World Health Day as "mental health," April, where "mental health day" and "health day" belong, was designated as "mental health month" for promotion, centered by mental health—related organizations. In the Mental Health Act amended in March 2008, Article 4−3 (Planning for Mental Health Projects) Paragraph 2, Item 4 of the project plan included the "awareness improvement project for mental illness" stipulated in Article 4.

6. Application of a Health Screening System Tailored to the Life Cycle

The national health check−up project in Korea is one of the successful outcomes of the health care system in Korea, which was implemented starting with the health screening for the insured by the Medical Insurance Management Corporation for civil servants and faculty in 1980. By providing major health screening services on a regular basis, it provided the basis for the prevention, early diagnosis, and management of chronic diseases. It has a variety of health screening systems that are unprecedented in the world to respond to the health risks of various population groups for the insured.

In accordance with the National Health Insurance Act, the national examination for health insurance subscribers is basically conducted for subscribers to the local medical insurance service over the age of 40 and dependents of subscribers to employee medical insurance. Examinations for employers are conducted regardless of age. This system has been targeting chronic diseases such as high blood pressure and diabetes since 1988. Since then, it has been providing preventive health management of diseases with the greatest burden of disease with the addition of the cancer screening program. The cancer screening project started with five major cancers (stomach cancer, colorectal cancer, liver cancer, breast cancer, and cervical cancer) in

1990, which has been expanded to the national project for early cancer detection since 1999.

Since 2007, the "Life Transition Health Screening" program for the 40−year−old and 66−year−old population groups and the "Infant Health Checkup" project for children under the age of 6 have been included. Health screening for the elderly is provided by local governments to recipients of National Basic Living Security over the age of 65 and those who wish to have a health screening for the elderly in the near poor class in accordance with the Welfare of Senior Citizens Act. School health screening is provided by the Ministry of Education in accordance with the School Health Act. Employee health screening is provided by the Ministry of Labor in accordance with the Occupational Safety and Health Act.

The elaboration of health examinations is leading to the development of programs that can manage health according to the life cycle—that is, health screening during the transition period and health screening for infants and children.

Life transition health screening has been implemented for those turning 40, "a period when the incidence of chronic diseases such as cancer and cardiovascular disease is rapidly rising," and 66, "a period when physical functions deteriorate and the risk of geriatric diseases such as falls and dementia increases (2007)." In addition to the general health screening, the 40−year−old life transition health screening includes tests for hyperlipidemia (triglycerides, HDL−cholesterol) and abdominal obesity (waist circumference) for early detection of risk factors for cardiovascular and cerebrovascular diseases such as stroke. Physical function (muscle strength, balance), daily life performance, cognitive dysfunction (dementia), and bone density tests (osteoporosis) were added to the 66−year−old life transition health screening[42].

In 2009, the "Framework Act on Health Examinations" was enacted to systematically reorganize the various health checkup systems.

7. Management of Public Health

Public hygiene services, which manage sanitation in workplaces used by many people, used to be managed under separate laws[43], and when they were incorporated into the Public Health Control Act in 1986, three sanitation−related services, such as laundry services, were added in addition to the existing four businesses.

Public health services are a service industry closely related to people's lives, and the industry has been differentiated to meet the needs of those who want more specialized services. Its management is also developing according to the characteristics of each industry.

---

42) 2012 Health and Welfare White Paper−Korea Association of Welfare Centers for People with Disabilities. [www.hinet.or.kr]

43) In 1962, the "Public Bath Service Act," the "Accommodation Service Act," the "Amusement Place Service Act," and the "Barbers and Hairdressers Act" were enacted and managed as individual laws.

Section 7

Promotion of Maternal and Child Health and Implementation of Family Planning

1. Background of Family Planning

After liberation, the population growth rate of Korean society was 1 to 2% per year. After the Korean War, the high marriage rate and birth rate led to a baby boom, resulting in an annual population growth rate of 3%. The total fertility rate was 6.0 in 1960, which not only continued the high fertility rate of the 1940s, but also caused social instability and poverty problems in urban areas due to the urban concentration of the population.

In the 1960s, the government recognized that the obstacle to economic development was overpopulation in the process of promoting the economic development plan and recognized the need for policies to reduce the number of children in order to escape poverty and reduce the burden of raising children. Therefore, the government adopted the family planning project as a population growth suppression policy as a national priority policy task along with the "First Five−Year Economic Development Plan" in 1962 and began to promote it[44].

2. Implementation System of Family Planning

The family planning project was carried out by a system in which the central government, city/province and city/gun/gu offices, ministry−affiliated committees, research institutes, and private institutions were all mobilized.

A. Government Agencies

In 1962, the government established an expert advisory system, established the Maternal and Child Health Division in the Health Bureau of the Ministry of Health and Social Affairs, and designated a department in charge of family planning projects in each ministry.

---

44) Ministry of Welfare, "70 Years of Health and Welfare" vol.2 Health Care, 2016.

As a regional project delivery system, "family planning counseling centers" were installed and operated in 183 public health centers (si and gun) across the country in 1962. As a workforce to carry out family planning, family planning agents were selected from among nurses or midwives and placed in public health centers across the country, and they distributed various contraception methods. In addition, the Korea Institute for Health and Social Affairs conducted research, investigation, and evaluation projects on health and welfare related to maternal and child health[45].

A family—centered health management system that comprehensively manages the maternal and child health project, family planning project, and tuberculosis control project was discussed, and this was introduced as an integrated health care worker system. In 1981, those who had been contract workers were converted into regular workers to ensure stable and continuous working conditions.

B. Population Policy Development Committee and Population Policy Committee

Despite the fact that the population policy was successful in decreasing the fertility rate, a number of tasks remained, such as family welfare, health maintenance, and stabilizing members of society. The "Population Policy Development Committee" was established with the goal of comprehensively considering these issues (1994). The committee decided to implement the "21st Century Population Policy Plan" from 1996 to shift the focus of the family planning project to family welfare. In the report presented by the committee, the necessity of policies for easing fertility control policies and enhancing women's social participation and rights was stressed.

C. National Research Institute

Family planning and maternal and child health projects are areas where policy formation and evaluation are made through research activities. In 1970, the government established the "National Family Planning Center." After that, it was given the status of an independent research institute, receiving financial support from the Ministry of Health and Social Affairs. This institution was for policy development through surveys, research, and evaluation for the efficient implementation of the family planning project by the government. This made it possible to cooperate with public health centers, which are the nationwide delivery system for family planning projects, research institutes that professionally and systematically support family planning projects, and city and provincial branches of the Korean Family Planning Association. This systematic approach brought about the success of the population growth suppression policy in Korea.

In 1981, the Korean Institute for Family Planning and the Korea Health Development Institute were integrated, expanded, and reorganized into the "Korea Institute for Population and Health," with the aim of conducting realistic and systematic research on the institutional development related to population and public health issues in general, as well as tasks in all related fields to contribute to the establishment of national population policy and health policy. Meanwhile, in December 1989, the

---

45) Encyclopedia of Korean Culture (Maternal and Child Health Service):
    http://encykorea.aks.ac.kr/Contents/Item/E0018543

research institute was expanded and reorganized into the "Korea Institute for Health and Social Affairs" in order to strengthen the research and research functions related to social security.

D. Planned Parenthood Federation of Korea and Korean Sterilization Surgery Association

Although the family planning project was carried out through the health administration system of the government, there was also a movement to actively and proactively promote it at the private level. In April 1961, the Planned Parenthood Federation of Korea was established, whose core business was family planning education and the distribution of contraception methods[46].

In 1975, the Korean Sterilization Surgery Association was established to actively deal with the adverse effects of sterilization.

3. Progress of Family Planning Project

A. Early Phase of the Project (1962 to 1971)

Family planning was established as a national policy in November 1961.

In August 1961, family planning training was conducted for 224 midwives, and the details of the project were reviewed at the "Conference on the Promotion of Family Planning Projects" in October. This conference developed into a "Family Planning Committee." Through active cooperation between the government and the private sector, the opportunity was provided for the Korean Family Planning Project to become a global success story.

After India, which adopted the family planning project as a national policy in 1951, and Pakistan, which adopted it in 1959, Korea became the third country to adopt the family planning project as a national policy.

The "Maternal and Child Health Team," established as a family planning organization in the Health Department of the Ministry of Health and Social Affairs, drafted the "10 – Year Plan for the National Family Planning Project," which contains the achievable population growth rate suppression goal.

The following is a summary of the major family planning projects by the government carried out during the period from 1962 to 1971, which laid the foundation for the family planning project.

---

46) In addition, the association launched the "Family Planning Mothers' Clubs" in 1968 to revitalize the operation of family planning projects and deployed 138 regional assistant administrators in charge of education on family planning in the county. A monthly "Friend of a Family" was launched in August to promote content related to family planning.

1961	· Abolition of laws prohibiting the import and domestic production of contraception devices : In the social atmosphere of the time, this was a groundbreaking event, and such a decision served as an opportunity to prepare for an epochal turning point in the spread of contraception methods.
1962	· Counseling centers set up at public health centers with family planning agents : Wide variety of contraception methods. · Training of family planners : Training was conducted for family planning agents in charge of family planning projects on the front lines and doctors in charge of vasectomy, a male contraceptive method.
1963	· Doctor training : The government conducted training for doctors in charge of intrauterine devices, a female contraceptive method. · Public health center instructors and community (eup/myeon) agents : 2,059 public health center instructors and community (eup/myeon) agents were deployed.
1964	· Adoption of intrauterine device (IUD) : It was officially adopted as a contraception method promoted by the government. · Introduction of the project goal system for each contraception method : The goal system is to allocate the project goal for each contraceptive method supported by the government to city/province and community (si/gun/gu) public health centers across the country, and even front-line family planning agents were challenged with the project goal.
1965	· Establishment and operation of a family planning evaluation team : For more efficient promotion of family planning projects, the necessity of conducting the project based on the accurate identification of the current situation and the measurement of the effectiveness of the project was recognized.
1966	· Operation of mobile surgery team : To provide contraception promotion services to the residents of rural areas (about 600 eups and myeons) with no doctors and to efficiently promote family planning projects such as contraception distribution, mobile surgery teams were introduced. · The "Three Children" movement
1967	· Deployment of maternal and child health agents : 152 maternal and child health agents were assigned to the rural areas (eup and myeon) to contribute to maternal health and the health of infants and children.
1968	· Distribution of oral contraceptive pills : As there was a phenomenon of avoidance of contraception due to the side effects of the intrauterine device, the government started distributing oral contraceptive pills with the support of the "Population Council."

B. Mid Phase of the Project (1972 to 1981)

In order to achieve the population growth suppression goal included in the "Third Five—Year Economic Development Plan" (1972—1976) and the "Fourth Five—Year Economic Development Plan" (1977—1981) for more stable economic growth, a stronger family planning project was promoted to counter the continued decline in fertility during this phase. The main family planning projects that the government promoted during the period of 1972-1981, the period of vitalization for the family planning project, were as follows.

1972	· Reserve Army Family Planning Project
1973	· Enactment and promulgation of the Mother and Child Health Act : By specifying that artificial abortion is permitted, the basis for legally implementing a family planning project to suppress population growth is laid.
1974	· Amendment of the Income Tax Act : Personal deduction limited to three children. · Introduction of menstrual control (MR) to the family planning project · Expansion of areas subject to intensive management of family planning projects : In order to expand the management target area from rural areas to urban areas, "Family Planning Centers" were installed in 20 low-income areas across the country, and access to contraception promotion services was improved in poor residential areas by deploying four to six doctors and family planners.
1975	· Industrial site family planning project
1976	· Industrial site family planning project : In order to diversify the available contraception methods and strengthen the project, fallopian tube surgery, a female contraception method with a high contraceptive effect, was disseminated. · Promotion of efficient distribution of male contraception methods : A vasectomy was provided through the military health center, and a male family planning publicity agent was deployed.
1977	· Amendment of "Family Act" for inheritance of women : The "Family Act" was amended, followed by diversified family planning projects such as urban family planning projects, hospital family planning projects, urban family planning projects, industrial family planning projects, population education projects, income tax exemption for up to two children, and corporate tax exemption for family planning expenses for employees. · Population education started in elementary and secondary schools : The population issue was added to the high school curriculum (social studies, biology, physical education, family, etc.), the middle school curriculum in 1978, and the elementary school textbooks (social studies, nature, physical education, practical subjects) in 1979 to expand population education to all school-age children.

1978	· Enactment of "Regulations on Housing Supply" : Priority was given to the sale of public housing to those who received sterilization with two or fewer children, and sterilization operation, the most reliable method of contraception, was promoted through the reduction of import taxes.
1979	· Distribution of condoms through cosmetic salespeople : As part of the condom distribution plan, condoms were distributed by cosmetic salespeople by signing a contract with Pacific Chemical and Seoheung Industrial Machinery.
1980	· Childbirth cost reduction system : childbirth cost reduction system for those who received sterilization after giving birth to two children in public hospitals.
1981	· Full-time health agents

C. Late Phase of the Project (1982 to 1996)

After the Korean War, the government pursued a stronger population growth suppression policy out of concern that the number of births could increase as the generation born during the baby boom period enters reproductive age. In particular, until 1985, the desire to suppress population growth had reached its peak, and the long−term basic goal of the population growth suppression measures promulgated in December 1981 by the "Population Policy Committee" was to keep population growth at the level of 61 million in 2050, and the total fertility rate at 2.1 people, the population replacement level by 1988.

This goal was actually achieved when the total fertility rate reached the population replacement level in 1983. Furthermore, from the mid−1980s, the fertility rate was maintained at a stable level of about 1.6 to 1.7 people. This fertility rate was far below the population replacement level and was lower than that of some advanced countries, such as the United States. The government, however, predicted that the population growth rate would increase if the fertility rate was not lowered as the baby boomers born after 1953 entered the reproductive age around 1980, thereby forming the reproductive age group for the next 20 years. Based on this judgment, the government continued to promote the birth control policy until the early 1990s.

Nevertheless, with the economic crisis, the fertility rate began to drop sharply in Korea, and the total fertility rate fell to 1.47 people in 2000. As a result, experts began to debate fiercely about whether to keep pursuing the population growth suppression policy.

In 1996, the government reduced or abolished the policies for suppressing population growth that had been promoted for more than 30 years, and completely changed the direction of the population policy to the "new population policy" to enhance population quality and welfare. Accordingly, in the 1990s, policies were implemented to dispel the problems expressed as male preference and artificial abortion, which appeared as side effects of the strong birth control policy.

The major family planning projects promoted from 1982 to 1996 were as follows.

1981.12	**· Announcement of new measures to suppress population growth** : Improvements to the business management system; the spread of contraception; the promotion of self-contained contraception practice; the reinforcement of the regulation and compensation system; the improvement of the social system; the correction of gender discrimination; the reinforcement of public relations activities, etc.
1982	**· Reinforcement of policies to support family planning projects** : Medical insurance coverage for sterilization surgery and intrauterine device surgery, priority support for housing funds and living expenses for those in the low-income class who received sterilization surgery with two children or less, living expenses support for those in the low-income class who received sterilization surgery with two children or less, free primary treatment for children under 5 of those who received sterilization surgery with two or fewer children, etc.
1983	**· Analyzing the results of population growth suppression policies and establishing future measures** : Supplementing support policies and regulatory policies for families with two or fewer children, the addition of free medical institutions for families of those who received sterilization surgery with two or fewer children, special livelihood subsidy for those in the low-income class who received sterilization surgery with three or more children, and restrictions on paid maternity leave for female workers with the amendment to the Labor Standards Act were included. **· Diversification of contraception methods** : Kappa-T, a female contraceptive method, started to be distributed. In the same year, the government established the "Contraception Management Committee" within the Korean Sterilization Surgery Association and began to take active measures to deal with adverse effects caused by contraception.
1984	**· Revision of family-related policies** : An amendment to the prohibition of hiring female seafarers to include the lineal ascendants of children who left the family within the scope of medical insurance dependents was made, and a preferential treatment system for single-child sterilization (under 34 years of age) families in the case of mid-to long-term welfare housing loans was implemented. **· Changes in the target of family planning project** : From the approach that was conducted for married women, the target of the project was expanded to include men in the reserve army in their 20s and 40s with strong fertility. Vasectomy was recommended for men who were participating in reserve army mobilization training. An institutional mechanism was prepared to let those who received a vasectomy during the training period return home after surgery and be exempt from the reserve army training for the year (five nights and six days).
1985	**· Preferential policy for families who practice family planning** : Medical insurance for dependents was expanded to include married women's parents, mothers-in-law, and fathers-in-law, and a free childbirth benefit system was implemented for single-child families. Policies to curb population growth, such as giving special rights to public housing to single-child families, were significantly reinforced. In consultation with relevant ministries, the "Medical Insurance Act" and the "Local Tax Act" were amended to prepare regulatory measures such as differentially levying medical insurance premiums and resident tax on families with three or more children.

1986	· Changes in family planning measures : The method of recommended contraception was changed from permanent infertility to temporary contraception. · System improvement : The livelihood subsidy for those in the low-income class who received sterilization surgery was changed from KRW 100,000 to KRW 300,000 for single-child families and from KRW 200,000 to KRW 200,000 for medical aid recipients. In addition, the "Mother and Child Health Act" was amended to provide a legal basis for family planning projects, and the foundation for the establishment of the Korean Family Planning Association, which had been based on the "Civil Act," was stipulated in the same law.
1987	· Amendment to the Medical Service Act : In order to resolve the imbalance in the birth ratio, the provisions for the prohibition of sex discrimination and the disqualification of doctors discerning the gender of a fetus were enacted.
1988	· Deployment of urban family planning agents : 200 urban family planning agents, five each at 40 public health centers in five metropolitan areas, were deployed.
1989	· Reduced contraception promotion : The government implemented a project to reduce the distribution of free contraception methods while expanding the distribution of contraception methods through the commercial network of private medical insurance. The free contraception methods were provided only to the low-income class and the disabled.
1994	· Amendment to the Medical Service Act : The punishment rules for doctors discerning the gender of a fetus were reinforced.
1996	· Relaxation of birth control policies : Changing the scope of income deduction for dependents, introducing priority loan measures for livelihood, farming, and fishing funds as well as priority for family welfare housing loans and public housing, providing civil servant allowance and tuition subsidies, abolition of restrictions on the scope of non-taxation of subsidies for education expenses, etc. Strengthening social support policies for women, provision of family allowances to married women's parents, and lineal ascendants being included in the scope of medical insurance dependents.

4. Maternal and Child Health Policy

A. Operation of a system for health management of mothers and infants

In 1963, it was attempted to prevent maternal death during childbirth by first hiring qualified midwives as maternal and child health agents. Due to the shortage of midwives, midwife licenses were issued to "midwives" (based on a decree of the Ministry of Health and Welfare, December 1951) who graduated from the "midwife training center" after completing a short−term course (six months to two years). This limited policy was maintained for ten years.

In 1967, with the implementation of the "Second Five−Year Economic Development Plan," 152 midwives were deployed as maternal and child health agents in the rural areas (eup and myeon) to provide safe delivery services. After that, due to difficulties in securing midwives, midwives at public health centers were replaced with nurses and nurse assistants trained through short−term training. Maternal and child health agents were responsible for ensuring healthy childbirth while implementing family planning projects. In other words, for those experiencing an unwanted pregnancy, artificial abortion was recommended, and those who wanted childbirth were registered as pregnant women. After childbirth, postpartum care was provided and the newborn was registered.

The maternal and child health projects included the vaccination program for infants and toddlers as an important program. In 1990, the vaccination program was transferred from the Quarantine Division to the Family Health Division and included as part of the maternal and child health program, as it was judged to be efficient to implement the vaccination program as part of the infant health care program originally provided. In 1966, in cooperation with the Korean Academy of Pediatrics, a vaccination schedule was developed to standardize the vaccination period for each type of vaccination, ensuring infants and toddlers receive essential vaccinations at the right time. As for the maternal and child health projects currently carried out by most public health centers and the projects carried out by leading public health centers, Lee Gun−se (2000) classified maternal and child health projects according to the life cycle into groups/organizations and communities, health promotion and management, disease prevention and early detection, health protection, disease management, other, high−risk, and special population. Accordingly, maternal and child health projects according to life cycle could be divided into three categories: first, existing maternal and child health projects; second, projects being promoted by leading public health centers; and third, projects to be developed in the future.

B. Laying the foundation for maternal and child health projects

After the Pharmaceutical Division of the Prevention Bureau of the Ministry of Health implemented comprehensive maternal and child health projects in 1948, public health centers were established as local enforcement agencies pursuant to the "Public Health Center Act" in 1956. In 1963, the Maternal and Child Health Division was established in the Health Bureau of the Ministry of Health and Social Affairs. Due to the reorganization of the government in 1999, maternal and child health projects were taken over by the Women's Health and Welfare Division of the Family Health Review Office[47].

---

47) Encyclopedia of Korean Culture (Maternal and Child Health Service):
   http://encykorea.aks.ac.kr/Contents/Item/E0018543

〈Table 2〉 Maternal and child health projects by life cycle

	Infancy	School-age	Adolescence	Childbearing age	Pregnancy	Middle-age
Group, institution, and community	Childcare and daycare facilities	School health	School health	Workplaces and business sites		Women's association
Health promotion and management	Nutrition and breastfeeding	Obesity, oral and sexual health	Smoking, drinking, and sexual health	Smoking, drinking, and sexual health	Prenatal care, pregnancy care, and health care	Nutrition and exercise
Disease prevention and early detection	Congenital metabolic abnormality tests, growth and development screening, early detection of disability, vaccination, and health screening	Health screening and eye examination	Rubella prevention	Rubella prevention and newlyweds health care	Gestational hypertension, diabetes	Prevention of cervical cancer, breast cancer, and early detection of osteoporosis
Health protection	Accident and disability prevention	Accident prevention	Suicide and accident prevention	Prevention of artificial abortion	Prevention of pregnancy accidents	
Disease management				Sexually transmitted disease management		High blood pressure management
Other	Management of children with intractable diseases	Children's health village and environmental care				
High-risk, special population	Registration management of disabled children and registration management of underweight children	Children in facilities	Child breadwinners and starving children	Single mothers and prostitutes	Intensive management of high-risk pregnant women	

※ Source: Lee Gun-se (2002), Strategies for Community Maternal and Child Health Promotion Programs according to Life Course, Maternal and Child Health Workshop, Ministry of Health and Welfare · Korea Institute for Health and Social Affairs.

In 1972, the department in charge of maternal and child health was upgraded from the Maternal and Child Health Department under the Health Bureau to the "Maternal and Child Health Management Office." The Mother and Child Health Act was enacted and promulgated as a separate law regulating maternal and child health.

The development of the Mother and Child Health Act, enacted by stipulating that maternal and child health was "to improve the quality of life by implementing appropriate health management during pregnancy, childbirth, and rearing to protect the health of the mother and fetus, and to promote healthy childbirth and nurture," led to the establishment of a pregnancy notification system and the reinforcement of medical examinations for pregnant women and infants in order to change into a maternal and child health business that reduced the mortality rate of pregnant women and infants through an amendment in 1985.

C. Maternal and Child Health Management in Medically Vulnerable Areas

Between 1981 and 1984, 89 maternal and child health centers were established in rural areas, which were medically vulnerable areas, and two maternal and child health centers were established in urban areas. One doctor was assigned to each center, and these doctors were public health doctors working in areas with poor health care instead of serving in the military under the Act on Special Measures for Health and Medical Services in Agricultural and Fishing Villages. Since performing only the primary care functions centered on general doctors and midwives was not sufficient to cope with abnormal delivery, there was a pressing need to secure a transfer request facility and to establish a comprehensive maternal and child health center by regional unit. With this system, the maternal and child health service delivery system was established in 1982. The main business functions of the Maternal and Child Health Center were maternal management, such as prenatal and postpartum management, as well as infant management, in addition to childbirth.

D. Measures to Improve the Quality of Maternal and Child Health-Related Services

The "Mother and Child Health Act" amended in 1986 required medical examinations for pregnant women and infants at public health centers. In particular, it was intended to protect the health of pregnant women and fetuses and induce safe childbirth by early detection of high−risk factors before childbirth. Where, health screenings for infants and toddlers were conducted at six months and 18 months of age, respectively, to detect and treat high risks and abnormalities early enough to minimize the sequelae. However, the capabilities and facilities of the maternal and child health personnel were not sufficient to carry out the infant health screening, and measures were taken to adjust the items and timing for the examinations. Although the examination items were not sufficient, it was meaningful in that it provided an opportunity for pregnant women to recognize the importance of health screenings by packaging the prenatal examination provided by the public health center and providing a comprehensive pregnancy examination.

In 1987, the "Health Risk Factor Table" was developed for comprehensive health agents to enhance the educational effect. After the "Health Risk Factor Table" developed by the WHO in 1978 was supplemented with content suitable for Korean conditions through pilot projects (Seocheon−gun and Asan−si), four types of health risk factor tables, including prenatal management, postpartum management, childbirth management, and infant management, were developed and distributed for nurses and nurse assistants, respectively. If the total score was higher than a certain score as a result of the assessment of the subject's risk factors, the integrated health personnel transferred the subject to a medical professional and requested it. The maternal and child health risk factor table primarily had the effect of educating the agents. In addition, it was used as a standardized activity guide tool to identify high−risk subjects and determine whether they should be referred to a medical institution.

Section 8

Changes in Policies for Disease Control and Eradication

During the Japanese colonial period, health policy was centered on hygiene administration. After the liberation, a new health management policy had to be established, and in the beginning, the introduction of the American−style public health concept was attempted under the administration of the United States Army Military Government in Korea (USAMGIK). The policy on the management of infectious diseases started with the establishment of the government in 1948, as well as the establishment of an independent health administration system. With the enactment of the National Medical Service Act in 1951 and the Public Health Center Act in 1956, the framework for national health was laid, but at that time, post−war medical relief projects and epidemic control were mainly carried out.

Since 1961, systematic national health projects have been carried out. In 1962, with the revision of the Public Health Center Act, public health centers were established across the country (si/gun/gu), laying the foundation for the implementation of infectious diseases and health care policies. With the enactment of the "Medical Insurance Act" in 1963, it was possible to create an infrastructure for health care organizations. Based on this infrastructure, the system and laws were reorganized in accordance with policy changes and disease patterns through the management of various water−borne and chronic infectious diseases, the implementation of family planning, the establishment of medical institutions, and the improvement in accessibility with the introduction of medical insurance. In 1980, the Act on Special Measures for National Health and Medical Care was amended to the Act on Special Measures for Health And Medical Services In Agricultural And Fishing Villages to deploy public health doctors and public health clinics to reduce the number of villages with no doctors, satisfying the quantitative aspect of the local health project infrastructure construction project.

The medical insurance policy that began with the implementation of medical insurance in 1977 was a monumental event that dramatically improved access to medical care through the implementation of the national health insurance system in 1989. As a result, the network of medical institutions and public health centers was expanded in response to the rapidly increasing medical demand. However, the expansion of medical supply and the stabilization of insurance finance delayed the introduction of preventive policies in public health policies for population groups and disease patterns, and rather showed the phenomenon of relying on insurance policies for health policies. Despite the fact that epidemiologic changes due to chronic degenerative diseases had already appeared in the early 1970s in mortality patterns, lifestyle habits, and economic and social aspects, public health measures began in 1995, with the enactment of the National Health Promotion Act and the Mental Health Act. In 2005, 10 years after that, the health promotion and disease prevention project began in earnest when additional financial resources were provided with an increase in the contribution of the Health Promotion Fund. In 2011, the mandatory vaccination for all children became a national support project.

In 1999, infectious disease management was transferred from the Ministry of Health and Welfare to the Disease Control and Prevention Division of the National Institute of Health. As real—time infectious disease information management was enabled through reporting system improvement and epidemiological investigation with the full revision of the "Infectious Disease Control and Prevention Act," evidence—based policies were implemented. As a result, the Korea Centers for Disease Control and Prevention (KCDC) were established with the successful management of the measles epidemic from 2000 to 2001 and the successful response to the SARS outbreak in 2004 to manage domestic epidemics and quarantine infectious diseases that cross borders. Infectious disease tasks such as vaccination management, AIDS, tuberculosis, quarantine management, and infectious diseases causing crises such as bioterrorism were newly established. Since 2011, when the budget for tuberculosis, the most infectious disease, and vaccine preventable diseases (VPD) has increased significantly, the "Disease Control Policy" was promoted into the "Disease Elimination Policy" (reporting, registration management, epidemiological investigation, vaccination and treatment expenses support, quarantine measures, etc.). Nevertheless, there is a high possibility that a new re—emerging infectious disease will be introduced and spread at any time. Infectious diseases such as bioterrorism in the United States (2000), SARS in China (2003), avian influenza in Southeast Asia (2003), the global influenza epidemic (2009), Ebola in West Africa (2014—2015), and MERS in the Middle East (2015) are infectious diseases of public health emergency international concern (PHEIC), which are infectious diseases that are a public health crisis task for which the world must quarantine and prevent the spread of inflows and establish prompt countermeasures.

Meanwhile, the Chronic Disease Investigation Division, which was newly established after 2004, enabled local governments to promote evidence—based regional health and medical plans, health promotion, and disease prevention projects through various health indices in their regions and evaluated the results by conducting regional health surveys and health behavior surveys centered on public health centers each year to evaluate various health projects implemented in si/gun/gu as well as cities/provinces. Continuous promotion of the 10—year cancer management plan, five—year cardiovascular disease management project, life transition period, and infant screening project was carried out. As a pilot project for chronic diseases, the high blood pressure and diabetes projects were also promoted in collaboration with Daegu City, and disease management projects such as asthma and allergy management in collaboration with the Seoul Metropolitan Government.

As the disease pattern in Korea has changed from infectious diseases to chronic diseases, advances have also been made in disease research projects. With the enactment of the Health and Medical Service Technology Promotion Act, the medical research and development budget, led by the Ministry of Health and Welfare, was organized by the

Health Promotion Fund. The focus of the research by the Korea National Institute of Health has also moved away from the level of internal research tasks, and full−scale research and development projects have begun. The modernization of the National Institute of Health and the relocation of government−run institutions to the Osong National Life Science Complex marked a milestone in health and medical research and development. The basic policy directions for health and medical research and development projects were established, and related medical science research projects were promoted in earnest with the opening of the National Cancer Center, the promotion of cancer research projects according to the 10−year plan to conquer cancer, and the reorganization of the Korea Institute of Health Services Management into the Korea Health Industry Development Institute.

1. Changes in infectious disease management policy

A. Changes in Waterborne Infectious Disease Policy

Diseases transmitted through water or food contaminated with pathogens, and representative diseases include cholera, typhoid, paratyphoid, shigellosis, and enterohaemorrhagic E. coli infection belonging to group 1 infectious diseases. These waterborne and foodborne infectious diseases are at the level of eradication due to the improvement of public sanitation and quarantine performance.

There seemed to have been 29 large−scale epidemics of classical cholera by 1940, and a significant decrease after 1970. Since the outbreak of 162 cases (142 confirmed cases) in Gyeongsang−do in 2001, there has not been a large−scale epidemic until now, and most cases are only sporadic due to inflows from abroad. In Korea, the overall number of infectious diseases has been decreasing due to the improvement of public hygiene and the development of the health care system.

In 1959, the gut microbiome office, which manufactured typhoid preventive drugs, cholera preventive drugs, salmonella diagnostic serum, shigella diagnostic serum, cholera diagnostic serum, and Widal/Felix antigen, succeeded in improving the manufacturing method of products with excellent antigenicity. In 1961, about 30 types of biological products were made possible, including BCG, typhoid, cholera, and smallpox vaccines, as well as tetanus and diphtheria antitoxin, and various diagnostic serums.

Cholera epidemics and sporadic epidemics continued as indigenous infections until the early 1970s but decreased sharply from the mid−1970s when public and personal hygiene improved, resulting in small−scale outbreaks of around 100 people. In general, there was an outbreak every 10 years, and the mortality rate reached 10%. Since the 1970s, the scale of outbreaks has not been large, and the mortality rate has also decreased to less than 10%. The risk of acute infectious diseases such as smallpox and typhoid, traditionally considered important diseases, has been reduced, whereas the importance of infectious diseases transmitted through collective food poisoning or overseas travel, such as cholera, Shigella, salmonella, Japanese encephalitis, and pathogenic E. coli, is increasing. The production of preventive drugs and diagnostic serums necessary for their diagnosis began in earnest.

In 1992, a total of 2,149 flights and 177,000 foreign tourists were tracked through a quarantine inspection of inbound travelers from areas contaminated with infectious diseases, detecting and preventing 11 cholera—infected cases from entering the country in advance. The possibility of the occurrence of a cholera group in Korea was very high, considering that it occurred earlier than the previous year, that it was showing a rapid increase, and that, in particular, there were four cases of V. cholerae O139 inflow.

Accordingly, the health authorities established special cholera prevention measures and conducted emergency quarantine work even during the winter season. The patient status and epidemiological investigation results were notified to the Ministry of Foreign Affairs and the embassy of the country concerned, and prevention promotion was carried out to overseas travel companies and guides through the Ministry of Transport. Efforts were made to block the entry of cholera into the country by providing on—site cholera testing training for quarantine inspectors for early detection of cholera.

In August 2003, the Quarantine Act was partially amended, and the new infectious disease syndromes, bioterrorism epidemics, and other epidemics of unknown cause were added to the quarantine epidemics stipulated as three quarantine epidemics: cholera, plague, and yellow fever. It was designed to properly respond to national emergencies such as severe acute respiratory syndrome (SARS).

With no cholera cases reported in Korea since the last outbreak in 2001, the cholera sentinel surveillance, operated mainly by the Infectious Disease Control Division of the Korea Centers for Disease Control and Prevention, has not been conducted since 2008.

The management system for waterborne and foodborne infectious diseases forms the basis of infectious disease management systems in all countries. Even in Korea, water—borne and food—borne infectious diseases were the representative infectious diseases that threatened public health before the 1970s, and they were managed as a major public health issue. Effective countermeasures were prepared step by step, such as a monitoring system that monitors the occurrence of infectious diseases, an epidemiological investigation for a group of infectious disease patients, and response measures according to the results of the investigation to conduct training for infectious disease management personnel, public relations activities to prevent infectious diseases, and quarantine measures to prevent the spread of infectious diseases. In order to monitor waterborne and foodborne infectious diseases imported from abroad, 13 quarantine stations nationwide are carrying out quarantine measures such as fever monitoring for those arriving from areas contaminated with infectious diseases[48].

B. Changes in Insect-borne Infectious Disease Policy

Malaria is an infectious disease that has been endemic since the past, which used to be referred to as "chills and fever." Since 1953, the number of malaria cases has decreased due to anti—malaria projects by the government and WHO as well as environmental improvement following economic growth. It was registered as a statutory infectious disease in the third group in 1963, peaked at 15,926 cases in 1970, and then decreased to a state of extinction (KCDC, 2014). In 1993, it reappeared as a soldier serving in the DMZ was infected with malaria. Since then, it peaked at 4,142 in 2000 and is gradually decreasing due to the active malaria eradication projects carried out by the government.

---

48) Ministry of Welfare, "70 Years of Health and Welfare" vol.2 Health Care, 2016.

In Korea, since the first outbreak of Japanese encephalitis was reported in 1949, large and small epidemics continued until the early 1980s. After 1,197 and 139 cases were reported in 1982 and 1983, respectively, no outbreak has occurred (KCDC, 2008). So far, the number of cases has been maintained at about 10 to 20 per year, almost at the eradication level.

In the 2000s, the Japanese encephalitis vaccination rate fell sharply to 54% in 2005 and 51% in 2006. From a policy perspective, this appears to be related to the lowered social interest in Japanese encephalitis and the revision of the vaccination schedule, such as the abolition of group vaccination.

As a result of this reduction in disease risk, awareness of vaccination has been lowered, and the inoculation rate has decreased since school group vaccination was stopped for safe vaccination, thereby lowering the level of herd immunity. In this case, a resurgence of Japanese encephalitis may be triggered by the vigorous breeding and growth of vector mosquitoes following global warming. Therefore, the Japanese encephalitis epidemic prediction projects, which had been maintained at 11 to 12 institutions, were gradually expanded to identify the trend and prevalence of patients to 30 institutions in 2006 and 36 institutions in 2007. This was aimed at early detection of the possibility of Japanese encephalitis, issuing a Japanese encephalitis warning, inducing vaccination, and ultimately minimizing the occurrence of patients by concentrating the quarantine agencies on mosquito control.

In addition, in 2014, the live attenuated Japanese encephalitis vaccine was included in the national vaccination program, and through various policies, the incidence of Japanese encephalitis in Korea has been maintained at less than 1 per million people since 1984.

C. Changes in Vaccination Programs

In 1895, with the enactment and promulgation of the "Vaccination Rule" as Internal Ordinance No. 8 of the Korean Empire, vaccination spread throughout the country. In 1912, vaccination was carried out with the production of a cholera vaccine along with a smallpox vaccine. In 1945, 18 types of vaccines, including diphtheria and tetanus, were produced and used through the Central Defense Research Institute, and in 1948, the BCG vaccine began to be produced and inoculated. With the enactment of the Infectious Disease Prevention Act in 1954, seven types of infectious diseases, including smallpox, diphtheria, pertussis, typhoid, typhus, paratyphus, and tuberculosis, were designated as routine immunizations, and the vaccination project was fully managed as a national preventive measure in accordance with the relevant laws (Centers for Disease Control and Prevention, 2008). In 1958, the first polio vaccine was introduced in Korea, and paid vaccinations started for some children.

In the 1960s, as vaccinations against typhoid, polio, cholera, and measles were expanded and distributed, the prevalence of infectious diseases in Korea decreased significantly. In the 1970s, vaccinations for infants and toddlers were expanded as part of the maternal and child health project, and in particular, the eradication of smallpox and polio during this period is a remarkable achievement. There have been no cases of smallpox since three cases were reported in 1960, and in 1980, WHO declared the eradication of smallpox worldwide (Centers for Disease Control and Prevention, 2013).

In the 1990s, as the "Standard Vaccination Guidelines" for infectious diseases to be vaccinated were developed and disseminated, the medical and scientific system of the national vaccination program was prepared, and universal vaccination services were established throughout Korea. In 1996, when the Mother and Child Health Act was amended, vaccination programs for all infants and toddlers registered at public health centers were conducted through public health centers (subcenters). As a result of amending the "Infectious Disease Control and Prevention Act", in January 2000, the basis for establishing the vaccination management system was prepared by classifying the infectious diseases subject to national vaccination as class 2 infectious diseases.

Since the launch of the Korea Centers for Disease Control and Prevention, the national vaccination program has undergone rapid development and service improvement. B Public services such as the hepatitis B perinatal infection control project (2002) and the introduction of the vaccination registration management system (2002) have been strengthened. In 2006, Korea became the first country in the Western Pacific to declare "Measles Eradication" by implementing large−scale vaccinations, monitoring infectious diseases, and strengthening registration management. In 2014, Korea obtained the "Measles Eradication Certification." National immunizations for children under the age of 12 have been provided free of charge through public health centers and designated medical institutions nationwide since 2014. As of 2015, in accordance with Article 24 of the Infectious Disease Prevention and Control Act, Korea has been dealing with diphtheria, polio, pertussis, measles, tetanus, tuberculosis, hepatitis B, mumps, rubella, chickenpox, Japanese encephalitis, Haemophilus influenzae type b, pneumococcus, typhoid, nephrotic syndrome, hemorrhagic fever, and influenza, which are designated and managed as infectious diseases subject to routine vaccination (KCDC, 2015).

In order to effectively promote the national vaccination program, it must be based on scientific evidence, and it is necessary to establish and manage national vaccination practice standards and methods. Therefore, the Vaccination Review Committee was first established in 1995 as an advisory body to the Minister of Health and Welfare in charge of the designation of infectious diseases to be vaccinated, cancellation of such a designation, standards and methods of vaccination, and review.

Also in 1997, the "Standard Vaccination Guidelines" for 13 infectious diseases (tuberculosis, hepatitis B, diphtheria, tetanus, whooping cough, polio, measles, mumps, rubella, Japanese encephalitis, typhoid, influenza, nephrotic hemorrhagic fever) were developed and disseminated Since 2005, "Standard Vaccination Guidelines" have been renamed "Epidemiology and Management of Infectious Diseases Subject to Vaccination," which comprehensively summarizes all aspects of vaccination and has begun to be published.

Vaccination is a representative public health project with high benefits compared to the cost of disease and death caused by infectious diseases. Vaccination has been proven to be cost−effective worldwide with reduced disease incidence and lower health care costs due to improved immunization rates. Therefore, vaccination is a part of public health management where a certain level of vaccination rate should be maintained by compulsory measures.

According to Article 24 of the Infectious Disease Prevention and Control Act, diphtheria, pertussis, tetanus, tuberculosis, polio, measles, hepatitis B, mumps, rubella, Japanese encephalitis, chickenpox, and other infectious diseases (influenza, typhoid, neonatal syndrome, hemorrhagic fever) require national vaccination in Korea. As the national vaccination coverage was limited to users of public health centers, users of private medical institutions had to bear the cost of national vaccination at their own expense. From 2014, the co−payment of KRW 5,000 was abolished and vaccinations were fully supported, marking an important first year for the provision of the national vaccination program free of charge.

The 2001 National Measles Eradication Five-Year Plan was to provide measles vaccination to elementary, middle, and high school students aged 8 to 18, who were likely to be infected during the epidemic, and to ensure secondary vaccination against measles in school-aged children. An active laboratory monitoring system was established to strengthen patient monitoring. The successful five-year project met the eradication standards suggested by WHO in 2006, and Korea declared measles eradication internationally.

In March 2014, the WHP Western Pacific Regional Headquarters Regional Measles Eradication Certification Committee certified Korea as a measles eradication country. In the evaluation of maintaining the eradication level after the certification of eradication in 2015, Korea was evaluated as continuously maintaining the measles eradication level.

The hepatitis B vaccine was introduced into Korea in 1985. Since it was included in routine immunization in 1995, the vaccination rate has improved, but the management of vertical infection, the most important route of transmission, was insufficient The positive rate of hepatitis B surface antigen (HBsAg) in pregnant women, which plays a crucial role in hepatitis infection, has shown a decreasing trend in the 1980s but has not shown a significant decrease in the 1990s, with a positivity rate of about 3.4% every year (Yeo In-seok, 2008)[49].

Accordingly, in June 2002, the government decided on a project to prevent hepatitis B jointly with the medical community. The "Hepatitis B Vertical Infection Prevention Project," in which the cost of preventive treatment is fully subsidized by the government, has been implemented since July 2002. From 2002 to 2006, 64,861 out of 70,183 newborns who were estimated to have been exposed to vertical infection with hepatitis B received support for preventive treatment. As a result, in 2008, the Korean hepatitis B management performance was recognized by the WHO Western Pacific Regional Office.

After a death case was reported from a Japanese encephalitis vaccination in 1994, Korea revised the "Infectious Disease Prevention Act" in 1995 and introduced the "National Compensation System for Vaccination Damage" for adverse reactions caused by vaccination to operate a system to compensate for medical expenses and provide temporary compensation for disability or death in the event of an adverse reaction due to vaccination.

In March 2000, the government computerized the monitoring system by introducing the electronic document interchange (EDI) reporting method. In addition, comprehensive measures to manage side effects of vaccination were established, and a dedicated organization was established to quickly respond to adverse reactions after vaccination, focusing on the national safety management system of vaccination. In 2001, the surveillance system was legislated by making it mandatory for doctors to report adverse reactions after vaccination (revision of the Infectious Disease Prevention Act), and in 2005, the surveillance system was diversified by introducing an Internet reporting system.

---

49) Yeo In-seok (2008), Summary of 60 Years of Korean Disease Control and Major Achievements, A history of disease control in modern Korea and its main achievements.

D. Management of Chronic Infectious Diseases Centering on Tuberculosis

Since the 1960s, Korea has established the foundation for the national tuberculosis management project through projects such as BCG vaccination and group screening. Since the enactment of the TB Prevention Act in 1967, the number of tuberculosis patients has decreased rapidly since 1968, but the rate of decline has been slowing since 2000. In 2013, there were 36,089 new cases and 2,364 deaths, and the number of tuberculosis patients in group facilities such as schools and military bases continues.

In 1961, the "Public Health Center Act" was amended, and since 1962, national tuberculosis management projects such as the BCG campaign and the home patient registration and treatment system were developed. Since 1963, one tuberculosis control agent has been dispatched to each of the 182 public health centers across the country. In 1965, with the cooperation of WHO, Korea conducted the first nationwide tuberculosis survey. As a result, the tuberculin−positive rate of those aged 5 or older without BCG scarring was 59.9%, and the prevalence of active tuberculosis was as high as 5,168 per 100,000 people. In January 1967, the "Tuberculosis Prevention Act" (enforced on August 1, 1968) and sub−rules were revised, laying the foundation for domestic tuberculosis management. A new tuberculosis department was established in the Health Bureau of the Ministry of Health and Social Affairs, accelerating efforts to reduce the incidence of tuberculosis.

Since June 2000, with the establishment and operation of a tuberculosis information monitoring system that allows doctors to report and track tuberculosis patients and physician patients through the computer, the National Tuberculosis Survey, which was commissioned by the Ministry of Health and Welfare and conducted by the Tuberculosis Research Institute to identify the domestic tuberculosis problem since 1965, was stopped after 1995.

As for the rate of tuberculosis incidence, which has plummeted so far, the rate of decrease has slowed down since 2000, and since Korea joined the OECD in 1996, it has consistently ranked first in terms of incidence, prevalence, and mortality.

The Ministry of Health and Welfare established the "2030 Tuberculosis Eradication Plan" in September 2006 through an interim inspection of the "Comprehensive National Health Promotion Plan 2010" in 2005 and presented the vision of "a healthy society free from tuberculosis." In addition, as the treatment of tuberculosis patients has gradually changed to the realm of private medical institutions, private−public cooperation projects have been promoted since 2009.

Currently, there are two national tuberculosis treatment centers in Korea: Masan National Hospital and Mokpo National Hospital In particular, Masan National Hospital is the only tuberculosis specialist training institute in Korea and a specialized educational institution for healthcare workers on multidrug−resistant tuberculosis designated by the WHO, which has a biobank in the clinical research institute. In addition, the International Tuberculosis Research Institute was established at Masan National Hospital in 2005 to establish an international tuberculosis research network under an agreement between the Korean and US health ministers. In 2009, it became an independent foundation and is currently conducting domestic and international clinical research.

One of the important goals of tuberculosis management policy is the early detection and prevention of additional patients through investigation of the patient's contacts for tuberculosis that is transmitted through the respiratory tract.

2. Changes in Non-infectious Disease Management Policies

A. Changes in Chronic Disease Management Policies Centered on Local Communities

From the mid−1980s, the need for chronic disease management began to emerge. Among the university−led pilot projects, service development through community diagnosis and a service delivery system centered on health institutions were established and began to focus on human resources development. In the early 1990s, projects focused on strengthening local power through participation in the local community, such as activating self−help groups using a wide range of information systems, were pushed forward. In May 1997, the Department of Mental Health was established, and the Cancer Management Department started independently in June 2000, providing an opportunity for the Department of Disease Control and Prevention to develop its main role in disease management. As a result, the Genome Research Center was established in March 2002, and the Korea Centers for Disease Control and Prevention received policy support through the establishment of the Chronic Disease Investigation Division in December 2003. Interest and investment in chronic diseases began to increase in the 2000s.

The Ministry of Health and Welfare set the year 2000 as the first year of the establishment of a lifelong health management system and introduced a plan to focus on improving indicators such as life expectancy, infant mortality rate, and cancer treatment rate to the level of advanced countries through the revitalization of prevention and health promotion projects.

The Ministry of Health and Welfare introduced the high blood pressure and diabetes prevention and management pilot projects centered on public health centers in 2000 and expanded them to public health centers across the country in 2003.

In March 2004, the Ministry of Health and Welfare included "establishment of a national disease control system" as one of the key tasks for the advancement of the health care system in the "Major Work Plan for Globalization and Localization of 2004." Accordingly, in June 2004, the "Basic Plan for Establishment of the National Chronic Disease Monitoring System" was established, and based on this plan, the monitoring system for the key management areas and indicators of the "Comprehensive National Health Promotion Plan 2010" began to be established. Since 2005, for the advancement of the national disease monitoring system, the monitoring system by life cycle, health behavior, and disease has been introduced in stages.

The Korea Centers for Disease Control and Prevention (KCDC) fully introduced the Community Health Survey in 2008, producing comparable health statistics between cities, counties, and districts every year, targeting adults organized by the Korea Centers for Disease Control and Prevention and conducted by public health centers across the country.

In 2011, the Korea Centers for Disease Control and Prevention (KCDC) started an activity to select the disease to be controlled and to specify the technical approach. Among chronic diseases, the major diseases with the highest burden are cardiovascular diseases, cancer, diabetes, and chronic respiratory diseases, which share common risk factors (drinking, smoking, lack of physical activity, and unhealthy eating habits), and diseases of the preceding stage, which can be addressed by a common strategy. As shown in the figure below, in 2015, the Korea Centers for Disease Control and Prevention (KCDC) set four lifestyle risk factors, four advanced—stage high—risk groups, and four major chronic diseases as key management targets, suggesting policy directions for them.

The Korea Centers for Disease Control and Prevention (KCDC) develops, produces, and provides evidence that guarantees effective chronic disease prevention services as a basic requirement for policy. First, the production and management systems of statistics for the national health and nutrition survey, community health survey, youth health survey, and cardiac arrest and injury survey were innovated. Second, the "Disease Prevention Service Committee" was formed within the Korea Centers for Disease Control and Prevention to establish a system for creating, reviewing, and recommending the basis for public health projects and preventive services. Third, priority research needs were identified in the field of chronic disease prevention, and evidence of chronic disease prevention and management projects was accumulated through research and development of effective preventive interventions. Regarding lifestyle risk factors, projects and strategies are being pursued, such as securing tobacco charges, expanding health promotion projects, reducing alcohol consumption, improving national nutrition, and strengthening campaigns to promote healthy living, which are described in the section "Active public health promotion."

B. Policy Support Direction for Rare and Incurable Diseases

Rare incurable diseases refer to diseases that have a low prevalence and are difficult to diagnose and treat with current medical technology. Based on the "Regulation on Designation of Orphan Drugs" of the Ministry of Food and Drug Safety, a disease with a prevalence of less than 20,000 or for which an appropriate treatment method or drug has not been developed is considered a rare and incurable disease. About 7,000 diseases worldwide have been reported as rare or incurable to date, and experts estimate that there are about 1,000 rare diseases in Korea. Rare incurable diseases are an area of market exclusion where diagnosis and treatment development are difficult due to their rarity and low profitability. There are many genetic and congenital diseases that often occur in infants and children and tend to become fatal or chronic. In many cases, there is no treatment or the treatment is expensive, increasing the burden of medical expenses. Due to the nature of the disease, access to medical services is low due to the lack of a professional workforce and information on the disease.

Since 2001, the government has started a project in which the government pays for out—of—pocket medical expenses, insurance equipment and wheelchair purchase costs, and respiratory aid rental fees for low—income people with four types of diseases: chronic kidney failure, hemophilia, Gaucher disease, and muscle disease. The Ministry of Health and Welfare has chosen the method of gradually expanding the target by discovering diseases that are subject to additional support. Afterwards, the Ministry of Health and Welfare continued to add diseases subject to special calculations through demand surveys and expert reviews and expanded it to a total of 138 diseases in 2009.

As for the case of rare and incurable diseases, it was difficult for not only patients but also health care workers to obtain disease information. Since 2006, the Korea Centers for Disease Control and Prevention have been operating the "Helpline for Rare Incurable Diseases" website (http://helpline.nih.go.kr).

The rare disease clinical research network supervised by the Korea Centers for Disease Control and Prevention has the primary purpose of collecting clinical information through observation of the natural course of the disease and collecting samples for use in R&D. By providing support for the analysis of special tests, which is not currently supported by health insurance benefits, the diagnosis and treatment of these patients is supported financially and technically.

In 2012, the "Rare Disease Gene Diagnosis Support Pilot Project" completed the development of genetic diagnostic methods for 17 rare diseases to enable patients with rare diseases to be diagnosed in a timely manner and take preemptive responses to diseases. In 2013, 11 diseases were added, and as of March 2015, a full−scale gene diagnosis support service is being provided for 28 diseases.

C. Policy Support for Cancer Management

As suggested at the "National Cancer Management Program Workshop" in October 1978 through technical cooperation with WHO, the cancer registration project began in 1980 as the basis of the National Medical Center hospital.

Korea joined the WHO's International Agency for Research on Cancer as the 17th member state in 2006 and is paying its share. Accordingly, research is being carried out in collaboration with the Scientific Committee and the Executive Committee.

Introduced in 2003, the "Cancer Control Act" developed a comprehensive cancer management plan as the duty of the government and stipulated the National Cancer Management Committee, cancer research project, cancer registration statistics project, early cancer screening project, and terminal cancer patient management project for dissemination and development according to appropriate treatment methods. In May 2010, the Cancer Control Act was completely revised, and the cancer information project, the central cancer registration headquarters, and the regional cancer registration headquarters were designated, and the guidance and supervision, and the designation of specialized palliative care institutions were supplemented.

In 1990, for the first time, the government established a "five−year plan for cancer management," and the establishment of the National Cancer Center contained the main contents. After that, reflecting the government's active will, the first 10−year plan for conquering cancer (1996-2005) was established. Emphasis was placed on the establishment of infrastructure for the prevention and management of disease and cancer. Therefore, the vision was to dramatically reduce the burden of cancer by minimizing the occurrence and death of cancer through comprehensive cancer management according to the "Second 10−Year Plan for the Conquest of Cancer (2006-2015)."

In June 2000, the Cancer Management Division was established within the National Cancer Center, which was established as a special corporation in 1999. The Cancer Research Institute of the National Cancer Center took over the functions of the National Institutes of Health Oncology Research Division. Thus, in May 2007, the Cancer Management Division changed its name to the "Cancer Policy Division," and in April 2011, when the organization was revised, the Cancer Policy Division was integrated into the Disease Policy Division.

The National Cancer Center planned to establish its own educational institution from the beginning of its operation, and in September 2013, the Ministry of Education received permission to establish a graduate school in accordance with Article 30 of the "Higher Education Act." In March 2014, the International Graduate School of Cancer

Science and Policy was opened.

As a result, the National Cancer Center has four affiliated institutions to support comprehensive cancer—related research, patient care and treatment, and the national cancer management project. The National Cancer Center has become the only model in the world that carries out comprehensive content as a project related to cancer management education.

With the establishment of Gangneung Calvary Clinic in 1965, domestic hospice palliative care started a general status survey of the pilot project for hospice palliative care for terminal cancer patients in 2003. Through institutional development from 2005, the designation of institutions in accordance with Article 10 of the Enforcement Decree of the Cancer Control Act began in 2008 based on the facility personnel of "specialized medical institutions for terminal cancer patients." In October 2013, the government announced the "Measures to Promote Hospice Palliative Care" to establish a specialized medical system for terminal cancer patients. First, "cooperative (advisory) hospice" and "family hospice" were newly established. Second, from July 2015, the daily flat—rate health insurance fee was applied to ward—type hospices. Third, in October 2014, by amending the "Enforcement Rules of the Cancer Control Act," the Minister of Health and Welfare exercised the authority to designate and cancel palliative care institutions. It also became mandatory to complete additional refresher training as part of basic training for employees of four hours every year.

Chapter 3

Discussion of major issues with respect to changes in healthcare policy

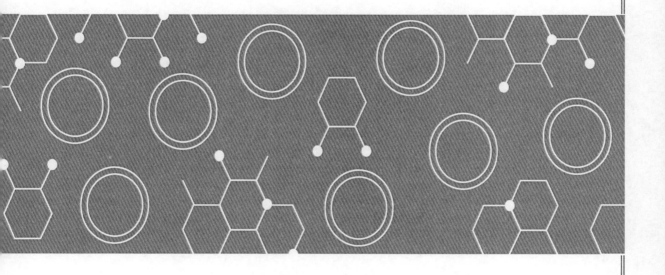

Section 1

Beginning of the Debate on Bioethics and Safety and the Transition Process

1. The Hwang Woo-Suk Scandal and Bioethics

For proper understanding of the Hwang Woo−Suk Scandal, which caused a massive shock and disappointment to the whole nation in 2005, an in−depth study would be needed across multiple fields including politics, sociology, psychology, and journalism, not only in life science or research ethics. This section aims to look into only the matters relevant to the Bioethics and Safety Act (hereinafter referred to as "the Bioethics Act"), which was enacted in January 2005. The main topics discussed in this section are as follows: the effect of embryonic stem cell research conducted by Dr. Hwang and his team on the Bioethics Act during its enactment process in 2004; how Dr. Hwang's research is positioned in the Bioethics Act that came into effect in 2005; how the revealed flaws of the same research at the end of 2005 were interpreted and handled according to the Bioethics Act; and what consequences the Hwang Woo−Suk Scandal had on the amendment process of the Enforcement Decree of the Bioethics Act after 2006. However, grasping the ethical issues of embryonic stem cell research is necessary for proper understanding of Dr. Hwang's research and the relevant laws and regulations, and therefore, an outline of the issues is provided below in the box.

Ethical Issues of Embryonic Stem Cell Research

A stem cell is a cell with the ability to differentiate into all kinds of cells such as nerve cells, blood cells, and cartilage cells in the body. Stem cells have been in the spotlight to turn the dream of regenerative medicine into a reality, which replaces or repairs the human cells, tissues, and organs to enable their recovery to normal functionality. For medical use of the stem cells, research on the mechanism of the stem cells to differentiate them into desired types of cells as well as the technologies of extraction and generation of stem cells with active differentiation ability are required. A group of stem cells that are processed to stimulate stable proliferation and to inhibit differentiation is referred to as a stem cell line.

Stem cells are categorized as embryonic stem cells and adult stem cells depending on the source of the cell extraction. Embryonic stem cells are derived from the inner cell mass of an embryo at the blastocyst stage. The advantage of this type of stem cell is that it is pluripotent—

---

the cell can be differentiated into all parts of the body. All stem cells that are not embryonic stem cells are categorized as adult stem cells. These stem cells exist in all parts of the body to make new cells to maintain health. Active research has been underway for medical use of the adult stem cells derived from sources such as cord blood, bone marrow, and deciduous teeth. In Japan, Dr. Shinya Yamanaka and his team at the Kyoto University successfully generated the induced pluripotent stem cells, which are considered as much pluripotent as the embryonic stem cells, by dedifferentiating adult skin cells to pre-differentiation cell stage by introducing several genes into the cells in 2007.

The embryo that is the source of embryonic stem cells can be fertilized eggs or somatic-cell cloning embryos made by nuclear transfer of eggs or fertilized eggs with the nucleus of other somatic-cells. The latter is particularly attractive because it can theoretically obtain stem cells that hold 99% or more of the genetic information of the owner of the original cell, minimizing the immune response when used for therapeutic purposes. The former does not have such advantages; however, fertilized eggs are easier to obtain than somatic-cell cloning embryos, and therefore involve fewer ethical issues as discussed later in this section, and securing sufficient fertilized egg embryonic stem cell lines has been reported to increase the likelihood of avoiding immune responses.

Embryonic stem cell research, unlike adult stem cell research, cannot avoid the confrontation of ethical issues. The various issues that arise can be categorized into four major categories as follows:

(1) Separating the inner cell mass that is the source of the stem cells inevitably involves destroying the embryo. This is particularly difficult to be accepted from the perspective of regarding embryos as life, and regardless of which point one considers the beginning of life, the possibility of embryos growing into life can cause controversy. This problem can be raised both in fertilized eggs and in somatic-cell cloning embryos.

(2) Another related issue involves whether embryos are allowed to be produced for purposes other than pregnancy. Article 23 of the Bioethics Act prohibits the production of embryos for purposes other than pregnancy. In the case of fertilized eggs, only the surplus embryos that have been used for pregnancy are allowed to be used for research purposes after more than five years, so this issue can be avoided for now. Somatic-cell cloning embryos, however, are obviously not produced for pregnancy purposes and can be problematic. If a somatic-cell cloning embryo is produced for pregnancy purposes, then the intention would be to clone humans, which can lead to 10 years or less in prison. Bioethics Act appears to have attempted to solve the dilemma in a way that does not view somatic-cell cloning embryos as "embryos".

(3) It is difficult to obtain the eggs needed to produce embryos and comes with a number of ethical issues. In the case of fertilized egg stem cells, they are also a step away from the problem of providing eggs for research, as they are producing embryos by fertilizing the eggs voluntarily provided for pregnancy purposes. As it was widely known from the Hwang Woo-Suk Scandal, the somatic-cell cloning stem cells research involves difficult ethical issues such as whether the providers received full explanation and signed consents, how to treat the case when specially related people such as families and researchers provide eggs, and whether to acknowledge the compensation for the provider, because the research requires to receive and produce large numbers of eggs for research purposes.

(4) Another important issue with somatic-cell cloning embryos is, as mentioned earlier, the possibility of opening the way for human cloning. A well-made somatic-cell cloning embryo,

which can be used for research and treatment purposes, can lead to the birth of a clone if it is successfully implanted within the mother body. No matter how strongly regulated by law and the researcher's conscience is firm, it is hard to deny that it is getting closer to human cloning, and as is commonly said as the "slippery slope", progress may accelerate in that direction.

While the fertilized egg stem cell research has problems regarding the issue (1), somatic-cell cloning embryos stem cell research has problems with all of the issues (1) to (4). In the course of enacting the Bioethics Act, agreements were reached between scientific and ethical communities regarding the fertilized eggs stem cell research, but not so much for the stem cell research in somatic-cell cloning embryos, and controversy continued after the enactment because the latter had bigger ethical issues.

A. Legislative process of the enactment of Bioethics Act and somatic-cell cloning embryos research

The first opportunity to raise interest in bioethics and even the need for legalization in Korea was Dolly the cloned sheep born in England in 1997, aside from the academic discussion of the need and possibility for bioethics distinguished from biomedical ethics[50]. As the possibility of the emergence of cloned humans as seen only in the movies has come closer to materialization, a series of bioethics regulation efforts began in July 1997, starting from Rep. Jang Young—dal's draft on the amendment of the Biotechnology Support Act, until the end of 2003.

The process of enacting Bioethics Act was, in short, whenever new issues were raised due to the development of life science, controversies surrounding these new issues sparked fierce debates and exchanges of public opinion, and all these eventually boiled down to enactment of relevant laws and regulations in the end. In this process, the association or logical link between the various issues raised to be covered by the laws and regulations was often obscure, and the Bioethics Act in 2003 did not have a comprehensive approach that encompassed development of biotechnology and its effect on human and the human subject research as well as the responses[51]. The issues discussed in the legislative process are outlined in the following table.

As the 15th National Assembly session expired in May 2000, several bills that had been waiting for discussion in the Science and Technology Committee and Health and Welfare Committee of the National Assembly were all disposed of. Then, the Ministry of Health and Welfare and the Ministry of Science and Technology took over the lead in discussion of these matters[52]. Around this time, Dr. Park Se—Pil at the Maria Fertility Hospital, Dr. Chung Hyung—Min at the Cha Medical Center, Dr. Yoon

---

50) About the overall Bioethics Act legislative process, see Hoon—Ki Kim, Biotechnology and Politics (Seoul: Whistler, 2005).

51) Bioethics Act was entirely revised in 2012 and has a separate chapter dedicated to "Research projects and protection of human subjects of research" to strengthen the nature of the Act as the framework act that aims to comprehensively regulate human subject research.

52) Hoon—ki Kim, pp.97.

Hyun—Soo at the MizMedi Hospital, and others succeeded in research to obtain embryonic stem cell lines from fertilized eggs. Dr. Hwang Woo—Suk applied for a patent in August 2000 to derive stem cell lines from somatic—cell cloning embryos[53], and he accelerated somatic—cell cloning embryos research together with Dr. Moon Shin—yong at the Seoul National University Hospital and No Sung—il, the Chairman of the Mizmedi Hospital. As the public's interest in the potential of embryonic stem cell research has increased, the ethical issue of embryonic research has also emerged as the hottest concern in the process of drafting the Bioethics Act by the Ministry of Science and Technology and the Ministry of Health and Welfare[54].

⟨Table 3⟩ Main areas of debate on inclusion in the Bioethics Act

Areas	Notes
Prohibition of Human Cloning	Included in the Bioethics Act (2003)
The permissible scope of embryo production and research	Included in the Bioethics Act (2003)
The permissible scope of somatic-cell cloning embryo research	Included in the Bioethics Act (2003)
Genetic tests, genetic information protection	Included in the Bioethics Act (2003)
Gene Therapies	Included in the Bioethics Act (2003)
Regulation on living modified organisms	Enacted the Transboundary Movement, Etc. of Living Modified Organisms Act (2001)
Patent of Life Science research results	Included in the Proposal of Recommendation of the Bioethics Advisory Committee of the Ministry of Science and Technology (2001) but concluded as an agenda to be covered by the Patent Act
Animal Research	Included in the Proposal of Recommendation of the Bioethics Advisory Committee of the Ministry of Science and Technology (2001) but concluded as this area was different from the human subject research's ethics and safety
Sperm and egg sales, surrogacy, euthanasia (life prolongation medical treatment), etc.	More relevant to biomedical ethics rather than bioethics. Prohibition of sperm and egg sales is included in the Bioethics Act (2003)

53) Hoon—ki Kim, pp.109.

54) Interesting part was that the debate at that time was active around how far embryonic research could be legally allowed, but there were no objections either from the scientific community or the ethics community as to whether embryonic research should be covered in the law. Although many countries were discussing the ethical issues of embryonic research at the time, few legislative cases were directly covered by the law. (Requires confirmation) The Bush administration's embryonic research guidelines (Insert explanation and reference), which had a major effect on the debates in Korea, aimed to provide grants to research meeting the guideline's requirements and did not prohibit the research even when they failed to meet the requirements.

The Ministry of Health and Welfare drafted the bill based on a research proposal entrusted to the Korea Institute of Health and Social Affairs, while the Ministry of Science and Technology established a bioethics advisory committee with members from all walks of life. Although the two bills were different in their process, they were largely consistent with the permissible scope of embryonic research, prohibiting the production of embryos for purposes other than pregnancy and infertility, and allowing limited research on the surplus embryos obtained for pregnancy purposes. In this trend, somatic−cell cloning research was not acceptable, and the scientific community and industry strongly opposed it.

In September 2001, the Board of Audit and Inspection proposed a legislative process in which the two ministries finalized the draft and consulted on it to determine the competent ministries. Following the proposal, the Ministry of Health and Welfare submitted a Bioethics Act draft based on the Korea Institute of Health and Social Affairs' research proposition, and the Ministry of Science and Technology abandoned the Proposal of Recommendation of the Bioethics Advisory Committee and submitted a draft on the prohibition of human cloning and stem cell research bill, which only regulates the core issues, to the Office for Government Policy Coordination. Both drafts took a more relaxed stance on the somatic−cell cloning embryos research. Therefore, the Ministry of Health and Welfare made the National Bioethics Advisory Committee decide whether to allow the research, and the Ministry of Science and Technology allowed the research but made the Committee decide the scope. While the scientific community generally accepted this limited research permission, the ethical community strongly protested and denounced the government.

In July 2002, the Office of Government Policy Coordination coordinated the two ministries to promote a single Act under the supervision of the Ministry of Health and Welfare, and after many twists and turns, a single government Act based on the one drafted by the Ministry of Health and Welfare was passed at the plenary session of the National Assembly on December 29, 2003. It was a moment when somatic−cell cloning embryo research was officially legalized in Korea.

B. Regulations related to somatic-cell cloning embryos research of the enacted Bioethics Act

Bioethics Act, which took effect in January 2005 after a year of preparation, was a substantially lengthy law consisting of 55 articles and addenda. Of these, the direct regulations of somatic−cell cloning embryos research were specified in Articles 22 and 23, and Paragraph 3 of the Addenda.

Section 3 Somatic-cell cloning embryos

Article 22 (Somatic-cell nuclear transplantation)
(1) No person shall engage in somatic-cell nuclear transplantation for any purpose other than research on a therapy for a rare or incurable disease under Article 17 (1) 2.
(2) The categories, targets, and scope of research that can engage in somatic-cell nuclear transplantation according to the research objectives under paragraph (1) shall be prescribed by Presidential Decree after deliberation by the National Committee.

Article 23 (Production and Research on Somatic-Cell Cloning Embryos)
(1) A person who intends to produce, or conduct research on, somatic-cell cloning embryos shall secure facilities and human resources specified by the Ordinance of the Ministry of Health and Welfare and file for registration of the establishment with the Minister of Health and Welfare.
(2) Article 19 or Article 21 shall apply mutatis mutandis to research on somatic-cell cloning embryos. In such cases, "surplus embryos" shall be construed as "somatic-cell cloning embryos."

ADDENDA
(3) (Transitional Measures concerning Research on Somatic-cell cloning embryos) Where a person conducting Somatic-cell cloning embryos research pursuant to Article 17, Subparagraph 2 at the time of this Act satisfies the following requirements, the person may continue to conduct research after obtaining approval from the Minister of Health and Welfare.
① Continued to research on somatic-cell cloning embryos for at least 3 years
② Published a research paper on somatic-cell cloning embryos research at least once in the relevant academic journal

---

Article 23 requires the provisions of Article 19 concerning the approval of somatic−cell cloning embryos research, anyone who intends to conduct somatic−cell cloning embryos research shall submit a research plan to the Ministry of Health and Welfare in advance for approval. However, while the scope of the surplus embryo research was explicitly defined in Article 17, The categories, targets, and scope of research capable of "somatic−cell nuclear transplantation" was to be prescribed by Presidential Decree after deliberation by the National Bioethics Committee (hereinafter referred to as the "Committee") in order to be approved in Article 22 (2). To get approval for the somatic−cell cloning embryos research: 1) organize the Committee, 2) pass the Committee review, and 3) be prescribed by Presidential Decree. Thus, first 26 cases of surplus embryo research plans were formally approved about eight months after the legislation's implementation, the approval of the first somatic−cell cloning embryo research plan would not take place until May 2009, as explained later on.

Paragraph 3 of the Addenda is a transitional measure considering that it will take time to organize the committee and a Presidential Decree is prescribed. At the time of the enforcement of the Act, researchers who had conducted research for more than three years and published papers in academic journals were allowed to continue the research with the approval of the Ministry of Health and Welfare. At that time, there were no other researchers who met these two requirements except Dr. Hwang Woo−Suk and his team, and Dr. Hwang obtained approval for the research on January 12, 2005, shortly after the Act was enforced. The requirement for paper publication was met in 2004 by submitting a paper on the first somatic−cell cloning embryos stem cell NT−1.

Therefore, researchers other than Dr. Hwang's team were unable to conduct somatic−cell cloning embryos research for some time. It would never be desirable for such a research monopoly to continue for a long time, not by the text of the law, but by a transitional measure. It was necessary to organize the Committee and obtain the Presidential Decree to determine the categories, targets, and scope of research of somatic−cell cloning embryos. However, due to the nature of the presidential committee, and the need to balance the selection of representatives of scientific and ethical communities, it took considerable time to completely organize the Committee and its five special committees[55]. In January of the following year, when the Embryos Research Special Committee came up with a draft of the presidential decree after much consideration, Korean society was already embroiled in the turbulent waves of the Hwang Woo−Suk Scandal.

2. Improving the Direction of Bioethics Research and Lessons Learned from the Hwang Woo-Suk Scandal

A. Outbreak of the Hwang Woo-Suk Scandal and the problems of research approval

After Professor G. Schatten of the University of Pittsburgh, who had been working with Dr. Hwang for two years abruptly announced his ceasing collaboration with Dr. Hwang on November 12, 2005, the public saw the myth of somatic−cell cloning embryos research fall from its peak into the bottomless pit over a half−year period until the prosecution announced the investigation result on May 12, 2006[56]. None of the 11 patient−specific stem cells, published in Dr. Hwang's 2005 Science paper, were

---

55) On April 7, 2005, the National Bioethics Committee was organized. The proposal of the five special committees was reported to the Committee and confirmed on October 10 of the same year.

56) About the whole cover of the Hwang Woo−Suk Scandal, see Hak−soo Han, *Dear readers, How should I deliver this news to you?* (Seoul: Sahoipyungron, 2006) and Yang−goo Kang, Byung−soo Kim, Jae−gak Han, *Silent Connivance and Public Enthusiasm* (Seoul: Humanitas, 2006).

found to exist, and even the NT−1 in the 2004 paper, which was known to be the first somatic−cell cloning embryonic stem cell, is highly likely to be the product of parthenogenesis. Even though more than 2,000 eggs were used, not even a single somatic−cell clone stem cell was obtained, and each and every abnormal behavior of the researchers, such as manipulating images, "mixing cells," providing researchers eggs, deliberations as a mere formality by the Institutional Review Board (IRB), and the repeated false statements, were revealed by the investigations of the Seoul National University, the Ministry of Health and Welfare, National Bioethics Committee, and the prosecution.

On January 12, 2006, when Science withdrew Dr. Hwang's 2004 and 2005 papers, questions were raised about the validity of Dr. Hwang's research approval a year ago. The research approval under the Act could be obtained only when the two requirements were met as seen above, such as continuing research for more than three years and publishing papers in academic journals. However, Dr. Hwang's 2004 paper no longer existed, and therefore, the research approval was now invalid from the beginning. The very regulation that enabled Dr. Hwang's exclusive research backfired as a threatening boomerang.

On January 23, the Ministry of Health and Welfare issued a preliminary notice of disposal to Dr. Hwang and other researchers under the provisions of the Administrative Procedures Act and requested to submit their opinions by February 10. Dr. Hwang and other researchers requested the suspension or postponement of the disposal decision, arguing that "substantive truth is under investigation regarding the derivation and maintenance of cloned stem cells, which are the source of the 2004 *Science* paper, and they are possible to resubmit or re−publish the paper." However, the consensus of the experts was that "resubmission" could not meet the requirements of addenda that required papers already published at the time of the enforcement of the Act, and that "re−publishing the paper" were even less likely to happen. The Ministry of Health and Welfare directly requested the *Science* to confirm that the resubmission of Dr. Hwang's paper was unlikely to happen and upon confirmation, canceled the research approval on March 16.

B. Subsequent direction of somatic-cell cloning embryos research

On October 10, 2005, before the outbreak of the Hwang Woo−Suk Scandal, the Committee referred the agenda of "the categories, targets, and scope of research to conduct somatic−cell nuclear transplantation" based on Article 22 (2) of the Act to the newly formed Embryos Research Special Committee and requested for a prompt drafting of the presidential decree on this matter as soon as possible. After three months of intensive work, the Embryos Research Special Committee voted on draft of the presidential decree at the fifth meeting on January 17 of the following year and presented the draft to the Committee on February 25[57]. However, the Committee

---

57) The draft of the Presidential Decree, which was proposed on this day, mainly called for imposing a number of ethical and safety restrictions (e.g. requirements for women who can provide the eggs and somatic−cells, number of sampling, consent) on the provision of eggs and somatic−cells, while several regulations regarding the embryos research of the Bioethics Act to be generally followed in the somatic−cells cloning embryos research.

decided to suspend deliberation on the draft presidential decree after discussions. Dr. Hwang's ethical flaws in the somatic−cell cloning embryos research were revealed, and they decided that fundamental reexamination of somatic−cell cloning embryos was needed at a time when the authenticity of the paper as well as the existence of the so−called "original technology" was unclear. The Committee had the Embryos Research Special Committee review the utility, etc. of somatic−cell cloning embryos research and submit the findings and opinion to the Committee.

Thus the reassessment of somatic−cell cloning embryos research began. The Embryos Research Special Committee was convened several times to perform meticulous probing on the matter, a discussion room was opened in BRIC, an online platform for life science researchers, and a joint forum was held between the Ministry of Health and Rep. Moon Byung−ho's office. Surveys were also conducted on bioscience researchers, members of the Bioethics Society, and the Biomedical Ethics Education Society. The survey attempted to ask whether to allow or support somatic−cell cloning embryos research by comprehensively reassessing various variables such as the research progress, economic feasibility of the research, ethical issues of the somatic−cell cloning embryos research, and other bioscience studies in Korea and foreign countries.

During the reassessment process, the difference in perspectives on somatic−cell cloning embryos research between scientific and ethical communities was still significant. The results of the reassessment reported to the Committee on November 23, 2006 by the Embryos Research Special Committee suggested a plurality of measures in light of these differences. The first proposal is a "temporary ban" that allows somatic−cell cloning embryo research after enhancing basic technologies such as somatic−cell nuclear transplantation yield and differentiation through sufficient animal research and fertilized egg research. The second proposal is a "limited allowance" that allows somatic−cell cloning embryo research under strict control. Specifically, the proposal suggested that the government should limit the eggs used in the study to "surplus eggs" collected from eggs that were not fertilized or removed, and to include the prohibition of transplantation of human somatic−cells into animal eggs allowed under the previous Bioethics Act in "prohibition of interspecies implantation".

After undergoing painstaking review, on March 23, 2007, the Committee voted for the limited allowance proposal without the members of the ethics division present, and an enforcement decree was implemented on October 4 of the same year. Bioethics Act, revised on June 5, 2008, included the prohibition of transplantation of human somatic−cell nuclei into animal eggs such as interspecies implantation. These regulations are the foundation of discipline in the somatic−cell cloning embryos research in Korea in 2015 when this book is being written.

<Enforcement Decree of the Bioethics and Safety Act (2007. 10. 4)>

Article 12-2 (Restrictions on Somatic-Cell Nuclear Transplantation)
(1) Research permitted to conduct somatic-cell nuclear transplantation pursuant to Article 22 (2) of the Act shall meet all the following requirements.
① Research for producing somatic-cell cloning embryos and establishing embryonic stem cell lines by using them
② Research using any of the following oocytes
   (a) Oocytes cryopreserved for producing embryos, intended to be discarded due to any reason, such as success in pregnancy;
   (b) Immature oocytes or abnormal oocytes, intended to be discarded because there is no plan to produce embryos;
   (c) Oocytes used for in vitro fertilization, intended to be discarded due to failure in fertilization or abandonment of fertilization;
   (d) Oocytes extracted for medical treatment of infertility, intended to be discarded because there is no appropriate donee;
   (e) Oocytes extracted from removed ovaries
③ Research using somatic-cell cloning embryos in vitro before the primitive streak appears during embryonic development.

<Bioethics and Safety Act (2008. 6. 5)>

Article 21 (Prohibition on Implantation between Different Species)
(1) No person shall implant a human embryo into an animal womb or implant an animal embryo into a human womb.
(2) No person shall engage in the following acts.
① Fertilizing a human ovum with an animal sperm or an animal ovum with a human sperm: Provided, That medical tests for examining the activity of a human sperm shall be excluded herefrom;
② Implanting an animal somatic nucleus into a human oocyte which is enucleated or implanting a human somatic nucleus into an animal oocyte which is enucleated;
③ Fusing a human embryo with an animal embryo;
④ Fusing human embryos with different genetic information.
(3) No person shall implant a thing produced from a procedure referred to in any subparagraph of paragraph (2) into a human or animal womb.

In December 2007, Dr. Hwang applied for approval of the somatic−cell cloning embryos research plan under the name of Sooam Biotech Research Foundation, but the Ministry of Health and Welfare rejected the application after the Committee pointed out the ethical issues of Dr. Hwang. It was in May 2009 when Cha Biotech was approved for the first somatic−cell cloning embryos research plan under the revised presidential decree. It was four years and five months after the Bioethics Act was implemented, and three years and two months after Dr. Hwang's research approval was revoked. In May 2013, Professor Mitalipov and his team at the Oregon Health & Science University in the U.S. made the world's first successful attempt at deriving somatic−cell cloning embryos stem cell line using the embryonic somatic−cell.

Section 2

Discussion on the institution of induced abortion

1. Background of the discussion on induced abortion and the current status

The issue of abortion has always been a subject of fierce debate in Korea. In November 2017, 230,000 people signed a national petition demanding the abolition of the crime of abortion, and the Blue House responded to the petition on November 26, "on this issue, we will conduct a survey on the current status of induced abortion, clearly identify the current situation and reasons, and based on the findings, the related discussion will be able to move on one step further"[58]. In addition, the Blue House pointed out that although the right to life of the fetus is previous and should be highly valued, the policy focusing on strong punishment has caused negative consequences such as the secret continuation of induced abortion, a myriad of illegal procedures, the burden of high cost of the procedure, going abroad to have abortion, and the risks in the procedure. The Blue House also stated, "the current system of laws and regulations places all liabilities on women, and the responsibility of the state and men is completely missing," and added, "In addition to women's right to self-determination, the possibility of infringement of women's right to life and right to health in the process of illegal induced abortion operation should also be discussed." In 2018, the Blue House further commented, "with the resumption of the survey and filing of constitutional complaints, the discussion in the Korean society will continue and the legislature will also undergo painstaking review on the issue," and added, "whether to legalize natural abortion inducing agents will also be decided based on the results of these social and legal discussions[59]. In line with the responses of the Blue House, on February 14, 2019, the Korea Institute for Health and Social Affairs conducted a national survey on induced abortion survey (2018) and presented the main findings. In line with the responses of the Blue House, on February 14, 2019, the

---

58) Nocutnews, Blue House, Answers the national petition on 'abortion crime'…"Start with the survey on current status of induced abortion operation" (2017.11.26.)
https://www.nocutnews.co.kr/news/4883030

59) Detailed survey results can be found in the reference added at the end of this book.

Korea Institute for Health and Social Affairs conducted a national survey on induced abortion survey (2018) and presented the main findings. This survey was the "national survey on induced abortion" conducted in 7 years since 2011, and was commissioned by MOHW's research contract service to Korea Institute for Health and Social Affairs in order to identify the actual current status of induced abortion using an online survey method and to understand related experiences of women. The survey participants were 10,000 women aged from 15 to 44 years, and the scale of the survey was expanded compared to the previous survey (2011) to ensure representativeness of the survey results and to enhance the accuracy.

In 2018, after 5 years and 8 months since the last one, there was a public pleading by the Constitutional Court of Korea in relation to a "constitutional nonconformity of abortion crime". This public pleading was held by the Constitutional Court of Korea for the purpose of reconsidering whether it is unconstitutional to impose criminal punishment to pregnant women who underwent induced abortion operation and an obstetrician − gynecologist who performed the operation.

On March 17, 2019, the National Human Rights Commission of Korea (hereinafter "Human Rights Commission") submitted an opinion to the Constitutional Court of Korea that the crime of abortion infringes women's basic rights and is unconstitutional. In the 4th Plenary Committee of the Human Rights Commission, it was decided that in relation to the submission of opinion on adjudication on constitutionality of statutes of Constitutional Court of Korea, the punishment of induced abortion is an infringement on women's right to self − determination, right to health/right to life, and reproductive rights[60]. As a result, on April 11, 2019, the Constitutional Court of Korea decided that the 'crime of abortion' of the Criminal Act was 'Unconstitutional' for the first time in 66 years, and it was ordered that the Crime of Abortion Provision of the Criminal Act should be amended by December 31, 2020 and if the amendment is not implemented by the specified time, the Crime of Abortion Provision will no longer be effective[61].

As can be seen from the above, the discussion of abortion in our society has continued to date, raising the necessity for reaching social consensus from various perspectives. Therefore, in this section, we will review legislation cases and precedents related to abortion and induced abortion operation and present an outline of the discussion. In the text, the terms abortion and induced abortion operation are used interchangeably. When using the terms in provisions such as the Criminal Act, the term "abortion" is used, and when emphasizing medical activities related to reasons for permission such as in the case of Mother and Child Health Act, the term "induced abortion operation" is used. In the Criminal Act, the term 'abortion' is used, and in the Mother and Child Health Act, the term 'induced abortion operation' is used. Abortion, also known as miscarriage, refers to natural or artificial expulsion of a fetus from the mother's body before the due date, or the death of the fetus inside the mother's body[62]. On the other hand, induced abortion operation refers to an operation to

---

60) Human Rights Commission, Criminal punishment on abortion infringes on the fundamental rights of women (2019.03.18.)
   The details can be found in the references added in the last section of the book.
61) Constitutional Complaint against Article 269 Section 1 of the Criminal Act, etc.
62) https://ko.wikipedia.org/wiki/낙태

artificially remove an embryo and any of its appendages from a mother's body at a time when the embryo is deemed unable to survive outside the mother's body[63]. The court definition of 'abortion' on Criminal Act is "artificial expulsion of a fetus from the mother's body before the due date, or the killing of the fetus inside the mother's body" (Supreme Court Decision 2003Do2780, April 15, 2005). Unlike in the case of Criminal Act, Mother and Child Health Act uses the term 'induced abortion operation'. In Article 2 Paragraph 7 of Mother and Child Health Act, 'induced abortion operation' is defined as "an operation to artificially remove an embryo and any of its appendages from a mother's body at a time when the embryo is deemed unable to survive outside the mother's body", and in Article 14, when there were reasons for justification, induced abortion operation is permitted. A brief description of the relevant provisions in the Criminal Act and Mother and Child Health Act is presented as follows.

2. Changes in laws and regulations in relation to induced abortion

A. Amendments in the Criminal Act

The provision in paragraph (1), Article 269, of the Criminal Act, enacted as the Law No. 293 on September 18, 1953, states, "A woman who procures her own miscarriage through the use of drugs or other means shall be punished by imprisonment for not more than one year or by a fine not exceeding two million won," and punishes the self−abortion of a pregnant woman. The provision of the paragraph (2) of the same Article states that the provision of paragraph (1) shall apply to a person who procures the miscarriage of a woman upon her request or with her consent, and paragraph (3) states that a person who in consequence of the commission of the crime of the as referred to in paragraph (2), causes the injury or death of a woman, shall be additionally punished. The provision of paragraph (1), Article 270, of the same Act states "A doctor, herb doctor, midwife, pharmacist, or druggist who procures the miscarriage of a woman upon her request or with her consent, shall be punished by imprisonment for not more than two years," abortion by the medical profession including medical doctors with the woman's consent was punished. The provision of paragraph (2) of the same article states that a person who procures the miscarriage of a woman without request or consent shall be punished, and paragraph (3) states that a person who in consequence of the commission of the crime of the as referred to in paragraph (2), causes the injury or death of a woman, shall be additionally punished. None of the above regulations stipulated the reasons for exemption of punishment.

As the Criminal Act was amended as the Law No. 5057 on December 29, 1995, the definition in Article 269 (1) of the Criminal Act changed from "a fine not more than 10,000 hwan" to "a fine not more than 2 million won", and "조산원(midwife)" in Article 270 (1) was changed to "조산사 (midwife; no difference in English)," and some phrases have been modified, but the actual content of the provisions remained unchanged.

Examining the current Criminal Act in detail, the Criminal Act stipulates the induced abortion operation as 'crime of abortion', and has two articles and seven paragraphs in

---

63) Article 2, Mother and Child Health Act (Definition).

relation to the crime. Criminal Act Article 269 (Abortion) and Article 270 (Abortion by Doctor, etc., Abortion without consent) stipulates the statutory punishment of crime of abortion as follows.

Chapter 27 The Crimes of Abortion

Article 269 (abortion)
(1) A woman who procures her own miscarriage through the use of drugs or other means shall be punished by imprisonment for not more than one year or by a fine not exceeding two million won.
(2) The provision of paragraph (1) shall apply to a person who procures the miscarriage of a woman upon her request or with her consent.
(3) A person who in consequence of the commission of the crime of the as referred to in paragraph (2), causes the injury of a woman, shall be punished by imprisonment for not more than three years. When a person causes a woman's death in consequence of the commission of the crime as referred to in paragraph (2), he/she shall be punished by imprisonment for not more than seven years.

Article 270 (Abortion by Doctor, etc., Abortion without Consent)
(1) A doctor, herb doctor, midwife, pharmacist, or druggist who procures the miscarriage of a woman upon her request or with her consent, shall be punished by imprisonment for not more than two years.
(2) A person who procures the miscarriage of a woman without request or consent, shall be punished by imprisonment for not more than three years.
(3) When, in consequence of his/her commission of the crime as referred to in paragraph (1) or (2), a woman is injured, such perpetrator shall be punished by imprisonment for not more than five years. When a woman dies, the perpetrator shall be punished by imprisonment for not more than ten years.
(4) In the case of the preceding three paragraphs, suspension of qualifications for not more than seven years shall be concurrently imposed.

The dictionary definition of abortion is to separate the fetus from the mother, the foundation of its life. Therefore, the general view is that the abortion is a crime involving artificial expulsion of a fetus from the mother's body before the due date, or the killing of the fetus inside the mother's body[64]. However, the Crimes of Abortion Provision is a legal requirement prescribed to protect the life of the fetus, but with the development of medicine, it was not possible to evaluate abortion simply as the artificial expulsion of a fetus from the mother's body before the due date.

Three legislative points have been raised to the Crime of Abortion Provision of the current Criminal Act[65]. First, there is criticism that it is unfair that the statutory

---

64) Lee Jeong−Won, Über die Struktur und die Problematik des Schwangerschaftsabbruchs − Im Vergleich vom Schwangerschaftsabbruch des deutschem Rechts, Journal of Legislation Research 54, p.193−216.

punishment of abortion by the medical profession with the woman's consent is heavier than the statutory punishment of crime of abortion with consent. The argument is that it is not reasonable to punish the abortion performed by a person with medical knowledge while engaged in medical profession more severely than that of a non−medical person. Second, the punishment levels are not in balance because the punishment of crime of abortion without consent is heavier than that of crime of violence, but the punishment of crime of death or injury resulting from abortion without consent is rather light compared to crime of death or injury resulting from violence. Lastly, there is an argument that the abortion should be discussed within a certain scope with the opinions in the direction of the amendment of the provisions, although this last point does not directly mention the problems with the current legislation.

B. Amendment on Mother and Child Health Act

Mother and Child Health Act was enacted in 1973 in order to contribute to the improvement of national health by protecting the lives and health of mothers and infants and by striving for the delivery and parenting of healthy children[66]. The Mother and Child Health Act, enacted as Law No. 2514 on February 8, 1973, stipulated permission limits for induced abortion operation. For the improvement of public health, first, the state or local governments shall take appropriate measures for the prevention of diseases and accidents for mothers and infants, early detection and treatment of diseases, etc. in order to promote the healthy development of infants and young children. Second, the permission limit of the induced abortion operation is prescribed. Third, it is to allow the government to subsidize the expenses required by family planning personnel. In 2009, the whole revision of Mother and Child Health Act was made. In particular, the allowable period for induced abortion operation was shortened from 28 weeks to 24 weeks[67]. Also, from the Limited Permission Provision, among eugenic or genetic diseases such as genetic schizophrenia for which induced abortion operation can be performed, diseases that can be treated or whose medical evidence is unclear were deleted, and the allowable scope of induced abortion operation was partially reduced.

The Mother and Child Health Act has a 'justification provision' for induced abortion operations for crimes of abortion under the Criminal Act, and Article 14 of the same law prescribed limited permission for induced abortion operation. Reasons for permitting induced abortion operation should be valid in medical, eugenical, or ethical terms. To be specific, medical reasons for exemption include eugenic or genetic mental disability or physical disease, cases in which the maintenance of pregnancy severely injures or is likely to injure the health of the pregnant woman for health or medical reasons, and she or her spouse suffers from any contagious disease prescribed by Presidential Decree.

---

65) Kim Young−Gon, The study of abortion law at legislative point of view, Master's Degree Dissertation, Graduate School of Public Health, Yonsei University 2006.

66) Korea Law Information Center, Reasons for enactment of Mother and Child Health Act. http://www.law.go.kr/LSW/lsRvsRsnListP.do?lsId=000183&chrClsCd=010202&lsRvsGubun=all

67) MOHW press release, Reducing the number of weeks allowed for abortion and prohibiting the establishment of postpartum care centers higher than three−story, 2009.04.03.

Infectious diseases due to which an induced abortion operation may be performed are German measles, toxoplasmosis, and other infectious diseases which medically expose embryos to high risk. Eugenic reasons for which an induced abortion operation may be performed are achondrogenesis, cystic fibrosis, and other genetic diseases, which expose embryos to high risk. Finally, ethical reasons for which an induced abortion operation may be performed are impregnation by rape or quasi−rape, and pregnancy between relatives by blood or by marriage who are legally unable to marry.

Under the conditions prescribed by the relevant laws, when there is 'consent of the pregnant woman herself and her spouse', a medical doctor may perform an induced abortion operation[68].

⟨Mother and Child Health Act⟩

Article 14 (Limited Permission for Induced Abortion Operations)

(1) A medical doctor may perform an induced abortion operation with the consent of the pregnant woman herself and her spouse (including persons in a de facto marital relationship; hereinafter the same shall apply) only in the following cases:

① Where she or her spouse suffers from any eugenic or genetic mental disability or physical disease prescribed by Presidential Decree;

② Where she or her spouse suffers from any contagious disease prescribed by Presidential Decree;

③ Where she is impregnated by rape or quasi-rape;

④ Where pregnancy is taken place between relatives by blood or by marriage who are legally unable to marry;

⑤ Where the maintenance of pregnancy severely injures or is likely to injure the health of the pregnant woman for health or medical reasons.

(2) In the case of paragraph (1), if it is impossible to obtain the spouse's consent due to his or her death, disappearance, unknown whereabouts, or other extenuating circumstances, the operation may be performed only with the principal's consent.

(3) In the case of paragraph (1), if the woman or her spouse is unable to express his or her intention due to any mental disability, his or her consent may be substituted by the consent by a person with parental authority or guardian, and if there is no person with parental authority or guardian, his or her consent may be substituted by the consent by a person who is liable to support her or him.

⟨Enforcement Decree of the Mother and Child Health Act⟩

Article 15 (Limited Permission for Induced Abortion Operations)

(1) Only those who have been pregnant for not more than 24 weeks may undergo an induced abortion operation under Article 14 of the Act.

(2) Eugenic or genetic mental disabilities or physical diseases due to which an induced abortion operation may be performed pursuant to Article 14 (1) ① of the Act, shall be achondrogenesis,

---

68) D.S. Kim (2014) Debates and Implications on Contraception and Abortion Policy: Focusing on Women's Reproductive Health Right.

cystic fibrosis, and other genetic diseases, which expose embryos to high risk.
(3) Infectious diseases due to which an induced abortion operation may be performed pursuant to Article 14 (1) ② of the Act, shall be German measles, toxoplasmosis, and other infectious diseases which medically expose embryos to high risk.

3. Changes in major court decision in relation to induced abortion

A. Decision of Constitutional Court of Korea on induced abortion in 2012

(1) Overview of the Case

Petitioner, a midwife who operates "xx maternity clinic" in Busan from around February 2009, was indicted based on the facts that she was commissioned to abort 6－week old fetus by a pregnant woman and thereafter, by inserting a vacuum device into the woman's womb and artificially eliminating that fetus out of the mother's womb, she made such pregnant woman miscarriage that fetus on July 28, 2010. While her case was pending (Busan District Court, 2010GoDan2425), the petitioner filed a complaint with the court to file a request for a constitutional review of Article 270 Paragraph (1) of the Criminal Act, under which the petitioner might be punished (Busan District Court, 2010ChoGi2480), to the Constitutional Court but that court denied such motion. Against that court's denial, the petitioner filed this constitutional complaint with the Constitutional Court on October 17, 2010, asserting that Article 270 Paragraph (1) of the Criminal Act violates the Constitution[69].

(2) Decision of Constitutional Court of Korea

The self－abortion crime in this case are adversarial crimes against the provisions of the law and, and since this case is to determine whether it is unconstitutional to punish a midwife who procures the miscarriage for a pregnant woman upon request, it was considered that if the punishment of self－abortion is decided to be unconstitutional, to achieve the same objectives, the relevant provisions of the law of this case that punishes a midwife who procures the miscarriage for a pregnant woman upon request are naturally deemed unconstitutional.

Examining the summary of the decision of the Constitutional Court of Korea, human life, the source of dignified human existence, is valuable so as not to be exchanged for other things, and thus, the right to life is the most. While a fetus has to be much reliant on the mother to maintain life, the fetus in itself is a living thing separate from the mother and, the fetus is very likely become a human-being, and should enjoy the right to life as well. Therefore, the matter of whether the fetus having the ability for independent survival cannot serve as the criteria for decision of permitting abortion. Meanwhile, if we do not punish abortion nor imposes sanctions other than criminal punishment, the abortion will prevail much more than the present state and thus the legislative purpose of self－abortion provision would not be achieved.

---

69) Constitutional Court of Korea2010Hun－Ba402. [m.lawtimes.co.kr]

Sex education, common use of birth-control method or support for pregnant women may be a means to prevent unwanted pregnancy, but these measures are not sufficient to serve as an effective measure to prevent unlawful abortions. Moreover, by allowing an abortion prior to 24 weeks of pregnancy in an exceptional circumstance including the instance where the fetus has mental disorder due to eugenic or genetic illness (Article 14 of the Mother and Child Health Act, Article 15 of its enforcement decree), the fetus' right to life may be restricted. Furthermore, the right to self−determination of a pregnant woman, a cause limited by the self−abortion crime provision, cannot be regarded as more significant than the public interest of protecting the right to life of the fetus through the above provision. Therefore, for the reasons above, the court determined that 'we hardly find that it is an excessive restriction on the pregnant woman's right to make a self−determination that the self−abortion crime provision does not permit an abortion based on social grounds or financial hardship, which makes such provision not violating the Constitution'.

Also, the court decided that the provision of the case prescribed an excessive punishment based on the following reasons: the upper limit is not so high because the statutory sentence should not exceed 2 year imprisonment; and, as for not so serious abortion crime, the court may make a sentence suspension or suspension of the sentence even it either does not reduce the sentence or has to make a statutory sentence reduction. Therefore, the court decided that they could not find that the provision did not comply with the rule of balance between responsibility and punishment.

Consequently, abortion is at high risk for depriving a fetus of a life regardless of the ways of abortion and most abortions are performed by healthcare professionals who have knowledge about abortion. Furthermore, they are highly likely to be criticized for performing abortions of depriving life because they are engaged in the business of protecting the life of a fetus. Moreover, considering that imposing a lenient fine on midwives seeking profits has a little deterrence effect, the court decided that they could not find that the provision where the legislature did not set forth any monetary penalty like the one for consensual abortion crime (Article 269 Paragraph (2) of the Criminal Act) was against the principle of equality violating the balance in criminal punishment.

B. Changes in the decision of the Constitutional Court of Korea on induced abortion in 2019

(1) Overview of the Case

The petitioner was indicted for performing 69 abortions upon the request or with the consent of the pregnant women (abortion by the medical profession with the woman's consent) (Gwangju District Court, 2016GoDan3266). While the case of the petitioner was still pending before the trial court, she filed a motion to request the trial court to refer the case to the Constitutional Court for constitutional review, advancing a primary argument that Article 269 Paragraph (1) and Article 270 Paragraph (1) of the Criminal Act were unconstitutional and a secondary argument that it would be unconstitutional to interpret the object of an abortion in these provisions as including that of a fetus within the first three months (Gwangju District Court 2016ChoGi1322). As such motion was rejected on January 25, 2017, the Petitioner filed this constitutional complaint against the above provisions on February 8, 2017 based on the same grounds.

* Constitutional Court Decision: Constitutional Nonconformity

① Decision on Self-Abortion Provision

The Self—Abortion Provision restricts a pregnant woman's right to self—determination to an extent going beyond the minimum necessary to achieve its legislative purpose. Thus, it satisfies neither the least restrictive means test nor the balance of interests test. Accordingly, the provision is unconstitutional, violating the rule against excessive restriction and a pregnant woman's right to self—determination.

② Decision on Abortion by Doctor Provision

The abortion by the medical profession with the woman's consent and self—abortion are adversarial crimes against the provisions of the law. Therefore, it was considered that if the punishment of self—abortion of a pregnant woman is determined to be unconstitutional, to achieve the same objectives, the abortion by doctor provision that punishes a medical doctor who procures the miscarriage of a woman upon her request or with her consent is also naturally deemed unconstitutional.

The Self—Abortion Provision violates the Constitution by, with certain exceptions set forth in the Mother and Child Health Act, compelling a pregnant woman to continue her pregnancy and give birth even if she faces the abortion dilemma arising from various and wide—ranging socioeconomic circumstances and by criminally punishing abortions procured in violation of the ban on abortion. By the same token, the Abortion by Doctor Provision, which penalizes a doctor who performs an abortion at the request or with the consent of a pregnant woman to achieve the same goal as hers, violates the Constitution.

4. Institutional changes on induced abortion

The examples of induced abortion legislation in Korea are the Criminal Act and the Mother and Child Health Act. The relevant provisions are the Criminal Act Article 27 (The Crimes of Abortion) and Mother and Child Health Act Article 14 (Limited permissions for induced abortion operations). As such, the legislation is dualized into the Criminal Act, which stipulates crime of abortion, and the Mother and Child Health Act, which stipulates reasons for justifications.

The decision of the Constitutional Court of Korea on abortion was made in 2012 and 2019. In 2012, the Constitutional Court of Korea ruled that the crime of abortion provision was constitutional. On the other hand, the 2019 Constitutional Court of Korea decided that the provision as the provision of constitutional nonconformity since it is an unconstitutional provision that infringed on the right to self—determination of pregnant women.

The discussion of induced abortion has shown the ongoing conflict between the right to life of a fetus and the right to self—determination of a woman's body. However, no conclusion can be reached through the discussion with these conflicting views. Nevertheless, in the midst of these difficulties, for a number of other countries, the legal system on induced abortion was developed as a result of drawing social consensus in various occasions of discussions surrounding induced abortion.

On April 11, 2019, in the Constitutional Court of Korea 'Case No. In 2017Hun−Ba127 Constitutional Complaint against Article 269 (1) of the Criminal Act, etc.', the decision was very different from the decision on August 23, 2012. In the 2012 decision, the provisions at issue in the constitutional adjudication was whether abortion by the medical profession under Article 270 (1) of the Criminal Act was unconstitutional, but in the sense that the constitutionality of self−abortion provision was actually decided in the adjudication, it can be regarded as the first historic decision on the constitutionality of the crime of abortion in the Criminal Act[70]. Meanwhile, in April 2019, the Constitutional Court of Korea decided that the 'Crime of Abortion Provision' of the Criminal Act was unconstitutional for the first time in 66 years, and ordered the amendment of the Criminal Act by December 31, 2020.

Now, in accordance with the decision of the Constitutional Court of Korea, the discussion of induced abortion in Korea should draw conclusions by December 31, 2020 on the following issues: determination of the period during which induced abortion can be performed, optimized solution for implementation between the protection of the life of fetus and women's right to self−determination, up to a set initial time, the period that induced abortion can be decided, including whether or not to request confirmation of social and economic reasons, combination of social and economic reasons, and certain procedural requirements (counseling requirements, deliberation period, etc.).

In this context, the legal system on induced abortion of major countries can provide useful precedents for implementation in Korea. In addition, the revision of the Crime of Abortion Provision of the Criminal Act has the special topic of induced abortion, and if social consensus can be drawn through interdisciplinary research with participation from not only scholars in law but also in ethics and sociology, it is expected that new amended provisions that can reflect the circumstances of Korean society can be prepared.

---

70) Jung Cheol, A Constitutional Study of Constitutional Court's Decision(2017Hun−Ba127) on the Self−Abortion under the Criminal Code, Korean Journal of Constitutional Law Vol. 19, Issue 2, Korean Constitutional Law Association, 2013, pp.324−325.

Section 3

Attempts to Introduce For-Profit Medical Corporations

1. The Controversy about the Permission of For-Profit Medical Corporations

A. The Current Regulations on Medical Institutions

Article 30 (2) of the Medical Service Act permits the establishment of a medical institution by a physician, the state or a local government, a corporation established for the purpose of rendering medical services, a nonprofit corporation established pursuant to the Civil Act or any special Act, etc. in, and Article 44 of the same Act prescribes that except as otherwise provided for in the Act, the provisions of the Civil Act concerning incorporated foundations shall apply mutatis mutandis to medical corporations. Also, Article 18 of Enforcement Decree of the Medical Service Act stipulates the mission of nonprofit medical corporations as to contribute to public hygiene and not seek profit (Oh Yeong—ho, et al., 2011)[71].

However, Article 2 (1) of the Foreign Investment Promotion Act[72] permits foreigners to establish medical institutions for purpose of rendering services for foreigners, and Article 23 of the Special Act on Designation and Management of Free Economic Zones[73]

---

[71] Oh Yeong—Ho, et al., A Study on the System Improvements of Not—for—profit Organizations (the first year), 2011.

[72] The Foreign Investment Promotion Act, Article 2 (1) ① and ⑥ b
 (1) The term "foreigner" means an individual with a foreign nationality, a corporation established in accordance with a foreign law (hereinafter referred to as "foreign corporation"), or an international economic cooperative organization prescribed by Presidential Decree.
  ⑥ b. The term "operator of establishments built to improve a foreign—investment environment" means any person who operates establishments prescribed by Presidential Decree, including schools and medical institutions for foreigners, in order to improve a foreign investment environment.

sets forth the provisions to support this, treating these medical institutions the same as medical institutions referred in the Medical Service Act. However, Article 5 of the same Act clarifies that these medical institutions shall not be deemed as a medical care institution established pursuant to the National Health Insurance Act.

As of September 2020, among all medical institutions in Korea that are the same or larger than a hospital, 51.9% (562 institutions) are established by nonprofit corporations and public agencies, while 48.1% are founded by individuals. Although their financial structure is in a devastating state[74] which requires reform, the institutional contradiction hinders it.

Analyses suggest that the debt structure is aggravating largely because its operating expenses are funded by short−term borrowing rather than a long−term investment. To make matters worse, the revenue of medical institutions continues to decline except in 2011. Low profitability is weakening their investing capabilities, reducing actual investment in facilities and equipment. Moreover, they have many limitations in terms of capital contribution. A low rate of return hampers capital accumulation; a difficult business environment limits the contribution by the holding company or the head of hospitals; the contribution with their own equity has no

---

73) The Special Act on Designation and Management of Free Economic Zones, Article 23. (Opening of Foreign Medical Institutions or Foreigner−Only Pharmacies)

(1) Notwithstanding Article 30 (2) of the Medical Service Act, a foreigner or a juridical person which is established under the Commercial Act by a foreigner, with the purpose of conducting medical practice, and meets all of the following requirements, may open a foreign medical institution in a free economic zone, after obtaining permission from the Minister of Health and Welfare. In such cases, the types of such foreign medical institutions shall be a general hospital, hospital, dental hospital, or convalescent hospital under Article 3 of the Medical Service Act:

(2) Any foreigner may open a foreigner−only pharmacy in any free economic zone after registering such pharmacy with the Minister of Health and Welfare.

(3) Where the Minister of Health and Welfare grants permission for opening any foreign medical institution under paragraph (1), he/she shall undergo deliberation and resolution by the Free Economic Zone Committee.

(4) Any foreign medical institution or foreigner−only pharmacy opened under this Act shall be deemed a medical institution or pharmacy established under the Medical Service Act or the Pharmaceutical Affairs Act.

(5) Any foreign medical institution or foreigner−only pharmacy opened under paragraphs (1) and (2) shall not be deemed a medical care institution established pursuant to the National Health Insurance Act, notwithstanding the provisions of Article 40 (1) of the same Act.

(6) Any holder of a foreign medical license, foreign dental license, or foreign pharmaceutical license may, if he/she meets the standards set by the Minister of Health and Welfare, work for a foreign medical institution or foreigner−only pharmacy opened in any free economic zone. In such cases, the holder of a foreign medical license or foreign dental license shall not render medical or dental services beyond the scope of duties permitted under Article 2 of the Medical Service Act.

74) Generally, state−owned and public hospitals are funded based on fundamental assets, while privately−owned and incorporated hospitals are funded by debt.

risk—sharing element; thus, it is almost impossible to attract investment. In order to overcome the current financial hardship and support and improve the public health, financial restructuring is inevitable.

B. The Concept and Attribute of For-Profit Medical Corporations

Before discussing whether or not to permit a for—profit medical corporation, we need to address what nonprofit and for—profit corporations are. In the legal definition, a nonprofit corporation refers to a corporation that does "not intend to make a profit," i.e., a corporation to serve nonprofit purposes, generally academic, religious, charitable, artistic, social, etc. Here, "intending to make a profit" is not intending to run a profitable business but pursuing profits for the members of the corporation, in other words, the personnel[75], and giving them financial benefits by distributing the corporation's profits. There are different types of the nonprofit corporation: incorporated associations and incorporated foundations established pursuant to the Civil Act and medical corporations pursuant to the Medical Service Act[76]. Unlike the nonprofit medical corporations, for—profit medical institutions can draw investments from outside, make a profit, and distribute their profits to investors.

Pursuant to the Medical Service Act, a medical corporation is nonprofit and not allowed to run a for—profit business except for medical practice, and only certain agents as prescribed in the law are permitted to establish a medical institution. In fact, a for—profit medical corporation cannot exist in the current law. The foreign capital can be invested only in nonprofit corporations, and under such circumstances, fruitage remittance is not allowed, all of which blocks foreign investment in effect[77].

Article 33 (2) of the Medical Service Act only permits agents to establish a medical institution as below:

(Article 1) A physician, a dentist, an oriental medical doctor or a midwife
(Article 2) The State or a local government
(Article 3) A corporation established for the purpose of rendering medical services
(Article 4) A nonprofit corporation established pursuant to the Civil Act or any special Act
(Article 5) A quasi-government agency prescribed in the Act on the Management of Public Institutions, a local medical center prescribed in the Act on the Establishment and Management of Local Medical Centers, or the Korea Veterans Health Service prescribed in the Korea Veterans Health Service Act

The establishment of a for—profit medical institution is not permitted under the current Medical Service Act. However, as foreign hospitals are opening in Korea and social awareness and structures are changing, the amendment of the Act should take the establishment of a for—profit medical corporation into consideration.

---

75) Personnel does not simply mean employees. It refers to the members of an incorporated association and shareholders of an incorporated company. (Source: http://oneclick.law.go.kr)

76) Korea Law Translation Center, http://oneclick.law.go.kr

77) Yim Joon, The Problem and Alternative of the Introduction of For—Profit Hospitals, The Seoul Economic Daily.

There needs to be a study on the form in which for—profit medical corporations should be accepted if they are legally permitted. We can think of various forms such as association, general partnership, limited partnership, limited company, or incorporated company. Also, for medical corporations for the public interest, we need to consider allowing them to render the service for profit partially, in some of their beds. That is to say, a hybrid type looks desirable to supplement the weakness of nonprofit foundations by permitting the public—interest institutions to establish their sub—corporation to pursue profit. This hybrid system can also be applied to for—profit corporations in the same way allowing them to run a portion of their beds for the public interest[78].

〈Table 4〉 Types of medical corporation

	Attributes		Types under the Commercial Act	The Proportion of Pay Bed	Remark
Medical corporation for public interest	Nonprofit incorporated foundation	Unification of existing educational corporations, social welfare corporations, etc.	Nonprofit foundation	5–10%	Tax benefit
Medical association	Established as a group practice	Group practice by 3-5 medical personnel	Association		
Professional corporation	Professional corporation	Medical personnel	General/limited partnership	Within 40%	
For-profit medical corporation (Contributed)	Incorporated company	Medical personnel (holds 51% or more of the share)	Incorporated company	Within 40%	

78) Park Min, A Study on Possibilities of Establishment of For—Profit Medical Corporation, The Korean Association of Medical Law Journal 9, no.2, Dec 2001.

It is evident without further explanation that the medical industry should fulfill the conditions of cost efficiency and profitability through the competition so as to adapt to a fast—changing health care industry[79]. In the United States, for—profit medical institutions take up 15.9% of general hospitals (the portion is especially high in a special hospital), and these for—profit hospitals can draw funds by various means of using retained earnings, borrowing debt, or issuing shares and corporate bonds (nonprofit institutions can issue tax—free bonds). However, if the medical expense, the quality, and the efficiency of the services they offer are better is still under study. In Germany, the majority of hospitals are state—owned or public (54.2%), followed by nonprofit hospitals operated by a religious organization (38.3%) and for—profit (7.4%). Investment in for—profit hospital chains is increasing with a positive review from the market. Although Japan bans for—profit corporations from establishing a hospital, the discussion regarding the matter is ongoing, albeit dividedly with pros and cons within departments of the government.

In Korea, as addressed above, all medical institutions are nonprofit corporations under the Medical Service Act, but when it comes to taxation, they are governed by the corporate tax law, which suggests that, from a commercial aspect, they are deemed as for—profit corporations in the Korean law. To reflect this on the reality and manage them effectively, private hospitals accounting for 90% of the whole beds should be given options to choose between for—profit and nonprofit corporation depending on the purpose of establishment and business strategy[80].

〈Table 5〉 Comparison between for—profit and nonprofit medical corporations

	For—profit medical corporation	Nonprofit medical corporation
The purpose of establishment	To provide medical service and make a profit	To provide medical service and fulfill a variety of purposes that are non-profit
The attribution of profit	The profit can be attributed to the members and investors of the corporation.	The profit cannot be attributed to the members and investors of the corporation.
Taxation	Governed by the same taxation with other for—profit corporation	Tax benefit
The disposal of assets when the corporation is dissolved	At liberty to dispose of its assets	Not at liberty to dispose of its assets

---

79) In advanced economies including the United States, commercial medical practices are generally allowed. It is understood that only a few countries including Korea, Japan, and the Netherlands prohibit the establishment of for—profit medical corporations.

80) ibid.

In the commercial law, as for−profit corporations share the same concept with ordinary companies, for−profit medical corporations will be allowed to fund capital, promote, improve efficiency for clearing debt, free from the pressure of acquisition of nonprofit hospitals, merger with other for−profit hospitals, have a less governmental intervention, and acquire and transfer shares. Moreover, they can provide patients with high−quality medical services by introducing developed medical technologies, scaling up the hospital, and funding greater capital to meet a variety of patients' demands.

The government actively supports and funds hospitals because their services are nonprofit and for the public interest. Considering a great influence on public health and care, for−profit hospitals should be established under the approval of the Minister of Health and Welfare, and at the same time, the government should increase the fund for public medical institutions to redress the imbalance of the resources so that all medical institutions perform their duty to help people sustain a healthy life. For example, nonprofit medical institutions in the United States are supported financially and materially including tax exemption, as well as a tax benefit to those that fit the strict criteria for nonprofit medical corporations in the tax laws.

C. Issues Related to Permission of For-Profit Medical Corporations

If medical institutions are recognized as a for−profit corporation, several legal issues are expected to arise concerning the mandatory designation system of a health care institution, health insurance, and advertisement of medical service. First of all, the mandatory designation of a health care institution under Article 40 (1) of the National Health Insurance Act needs to be reviewed since it would restrict the diversification of for−profit corporations' business operations. Also, the introduction of private insurance should be closely examined to address the problems of the medical fee paid by health insurance. For the matter of diversifying medical services, we need to consider the introduction of private insurance and make sure that its coverage does not overlap with the national health insurance (NHI). Furthermore, the regulations on medical advertisement should be amended.

Also, an in−depth study should be preceded with a prerequisite that a number of problems can arise from transferring hospitals from nonprofit to for−profit, followed by legislation to apply to the process of opening for−profit medical corporations, e.g., hospital chains or merger and acquisition.

2. The Major Issue and the History of Discussion

A. The History of the Controversy

In Korea, the introduction of for−profit medical corporations was first discussed in 1995, coupled with the agenda of opening the health care market, aiming to enhance the competitiveness of the field. Since the amendment of law permitted the establishment of for−profit hospitals and medical practice for Koreans in free economic zones including Songdo in Incheon, the government began to propose to legalize for−profit hospitals on a nationwide scale[81]. Backed by this movement, large private hospitals and insurance carriers strongly called for the introduction of for−profit medical corporations for more developed and competitive medical services[82]. In February 2006, the permission of a foreign−invested for−profit medical corporation was granted in Jeju Island, and in October 2009, the Ministry of Health and Welfare announced that it would approve the request for the opening of domestically−invested medical corporations.

The enactment of the Special Act on the Establishment of Jeju Special Self−Governing Province permitted the establishment of foreign for−profit hospitals that can conduct medical practice for Koreans. Furthermore, the government tried to open the Korean health care market by allowing advertisement and subsidiary business operation, etc[83]. Led by the enactment and amendment of the special act for for−profit hospitals, the bill to amend the Medical Service Act had been suggested to partially allow hospitals to invite patients or recommend medical services but was scrapped in 2007. In conclusion, the Korean government fundamentally prohibits the establishment and operation of for−profit medical corporations except for some special cases in free economic zones and Jeju Island.

The debate between advocates and opponents is ongoing in various fields of Korean society, and no one can predict the consequence. The new administration that started in 2013 announced that it would permit the establishment of for−profit hospitals and medical practices for Koreans in free economic zones, following the Lee Myung−Bak administration's policy to privatize the country's healthcare system. However, since the privatization policy is facing strong opposition from health−care−related civic groups, we will have to wait and see how the policy will be pushed forward together with the amendment of relevant laws[84].

---

81) Yim Joon, The Problem and Alternative of the Introduction of For−Profit Hospitals, The Seoul Economic Daily.

82) Park Seung−ju, Are For−Profit Hospitals Good This Way?, Health Right Network.
[Dated: October 01, 2013]
http://www.konkang21.or.kr/bbs/board.php?bo_table=free&wr_id=22614&sfl=wr_subject&stx=&sst=wr_last&sod=desc&sop=and&page=37

83) Yim Joon, The Problem and Alternative of the Introduction of For−Profit Hospitals, The Seoul Economic Daily.

84) Lee Hyo−Jeong, Civic Groups Put the Brakes on President−Elect Lee's Health Care Privatization, Medipana. (December 27, 2012) [Dated online: October 01, 2013]
http://medipana.com/news/news_viewer.asp?NewsNum=100535&MainKind =A&NewsKind=5&vCount=12&vKind=1

B. The Major Issue

The advocates claim that for−profit hospitals have the following advantages: First, the competition with for−profit hospitals and private insurance carriers will improve the quality of medical services. Second, hospitals will be able to draw investment. Third, medical services will become diversified to meet the market expectation. Fourth, high−end services will help attract foreign patients and contribute to the nation's wealth (Yu In−Mo, Kim Ki−Chan, 2008).

On the contrary, the opponents refute with the following reasons: First, since the hospital revenue is not large in the first place, it will not be of a significant help for investment attraction. Second, the free competition might lower the quality of medical practice rather than improving it. Third, it is difficult to estimate the demands of patients going abroad for high−end service or determine whether they are genuinely seeking after high−end service and it is also difficult to present the evidence for to what extent the domestic medical practice should be upgraded to prevent this trend. Fourth, although some advanced countries permit for−profit hospitals, in practice, few hospitals become for−profit. Fifth, medical expenses are expected to increase. Sixth, it can shake the foundation and perpetuity of the healthcare system (Gam Shin, 2004).

The problem facing the Korean government's policymaking is that the issue more often than not sparks ideological clashes, unable to be discussed based on empirical data. Despite overwhelming concerns about rising medical expense when introducing a for−profit corporation, there hasn't been a consumer survey or a study on changes of medical service use according to rising medical fees by suggesting a specific condition of fee and service, e.g., whether consumers intend to use the service even if the fee rises by 10 percent.

In 2004 and 2005, under the Roh Moo−Hyun administration, the subject became controversial as the president and the Ministry of Health and Welfare had different stances, making it difficult to set a practical policy direction. Since the Ministry had been reviewing the agenda from the opponents' perspective, it had very little empirical data investigated from the neutral aspect to anticipate what will happen when introducing the policy. The Korean Health Industry Development Institute (KHIDI) and other researchers also said it is not desirable to study without having a concrete stance. In the end, the Ministry failed to suggest any empirical data regarding its impact on the economy.

In 2008 and 2009, the issue was highlighted once again. The Ministry of Economy and Finance argued that for−profit medical corporations will boost the nation's health care industry shortly. On the other hand, the Ministry of Health and Welfare, the department practically in charge of this issue, refuted that what the Ministry of Economy and Finance predicts is not likely to happen and there will be drawbacks more than benefits. However, both argued based on summarized foreign case studies without any practical verification of its effect. Indeed, there were arguments but not any empirical data.

Then−president Lee Myung−Bak tried to introduce incorporated for−profit medical institutions. However, in the early days, his administration faced a backlash against American beef imports, and liberals attempted to move and continue the controversy on the for−profit medical corporation issue. Fueled by an American documentary film Sicko that gained popularity, the liberals argued, if the government introduces the concept of a for−profit medical corporation, the Korean healthcare system would become like the foreign one. This put the government in a difficult position. The issue was a key national agenda, so it could not be dismissed, nor could it be pushed ahead due to the burden from other national affairs. Hence, it was proposed to conduct empirical verification of the impact of the policy.

The Ministry of Economy and Finance commissioned the Korea Development Institute (KDI) to study its impact on the health care industry, while the Ministry of Health and Welfare commissioned the Korea Institute for Health and Social Affairs (KIHASA) to investigate the possible problems. The reports were released after six months of research, in which KDI laid out somewhat banal conclusion without specific estimates, citing the current and future rankings of the health industry just as it was previously argued, whereas KIHASA presented more specific results but still short of empirical data (see the reports released in 2009 by KIHASA and KDI).

Some are concerned that, if for−profit hospitals are introduced, they will be excluded from the mandatory designation system of health insurance, which would disturb the NHI system severely. In other words, patients of for−profit hospitals, who are likely to be relatively affluent, will pay expensive medical fees at their own expense or will be insured privately.

Then, the private insurer will apply the same amount of medical fee and the fee system with that of NHI to for−profit hospitals, and those hospitals will provide the service mainly for those privately insured from whom they can get paid and in essence, these hospitals will become inaccessible to NHI policyholders. This would divide the medical institutions into two by the income of patients: for−profit hospitals that provide luxurious service for expensive private insurance policyholders and nonprofit hospitals that provide ordinary service for national insurance policyholders and patients with medical care, exacerbating inequality in terms of using health care service.

Nevertheless, such concerns can be dealt with differently depending on a policy decision, e.g., how the mandatory designation system or the payment of medical fees should be applied to for−profit hospitals. Unfortunately, the Korean government has maintained the same policy that it would examine the accomplishment after building open−type hospitals in free economic zones including Jeju and Incheon.

For−profit hospitals in the free economic zone in Incheon were actually planned not to be covered by health insurance even for Korean patients. However, this was forecasted to cause difficulties in operating the hospitals because it is likely to decline the numer of patients and increase fees. Therefore, they were designed to be covered by the health insurance, as well as in a way to promote the use by Korean patients.

The introduction of a subsidiary corporation, one of the latest issues, has a different context from the introduction of a for−profit medical corporation as the former is about establishing for−profit subsidiaries of medical corporations within the limited scope. For instance, nonprofit corporations such as a school or a social welfare center can establish a for−profit subsidiary, which might be used to argue that this permission should also be applied to nonprofit medical corporations. However, in the case of a nonprofit school or welfare center, only a restricted percentage of its revenue lawfully earned for the purpose of establishment is permitted to be spent for other purposes. Besides, the for−profit subsidiary concept is fundamentally different from that of a for−profit medical corporation. A significant distinction between for−profit and nonprofit medical corporations lies in whether it can invite investment at its discretion and the income is permitted to inure to the benefit of investors.

The UK government provided tax benefits for private health insurance policyholders during the reform of the National Health Service (NHS) in the early 1990s, which triggered a debate in the country that values fairness in terms of policymaking. In the end, the government decided that private insurance policyholders should stay in the NHS and allowed them to use for−profit hospitals instead of the NHS hospitals so that it can help support the finance of NHS. Nevertheless, few people bought private insurance. Instead, companies took it out for employees as one of the employee benefits. The company paid the premium, and employees could use it at once when they go to a for−profit hospital. Still, private health insurance policyholders did not exceed 11% of the entire population (based on the past data). The demand was very limited. The Netherlands also gives an option for people to take out private health insurance as an alternative to its universal social health insurance, but in fact, it is also limitedly chosen by some of the affluent. Liberal groups in Korea condemn for−profit hospitals that they will polarize the healthcare system. However, the case of the United Kingdom shows that its expansion is limited. Of course, the coverages are different, but we need to give some time to think about it.

Another concern is that, if the premium rises, people with high income might use health care services more. In general, a high−income bracket uses medical services more. Even if the premium section of the health insurance system is designed fairly, there is a risk that a high−income bracket might take more portion of the service. If we allow people to hold both the national and private health insurance like the NHS system in the UK, it might increase the financial soundness of NHI.

C. The Concept of Pay Bed

In 1995 and 1996, under President Kim Young−Sam, the health care reform committee reflected the process of meeting or proposals on the policy including the resource−based relative value scale (RBRVS) and the diagnosis related group (DRG). The final report served as a guideline of policy direction for the Ministry of Health and Welfare, which includes the proposal to run beds not covered by the insurance.

It pointed out that one of the reasons why the affluent go overseas for medical treatment is a low satisfaction with the service quality under the NHI system, so why not allow them to pay all medical fees at their own expenses if they want a bed not covered by the national insurance, even if they hold NHI or their illness is subject to be covered by NHI. This would increase patients' satisfaction and also enable a hospital to practice more advanced medical techniques. In doing so, it will fulfill the needs of physicians to develop medical techniques and reduce the expenditure on health insurance.

This concept is called pay bed in the United Kingdom, and a positive examination was necessary to introduce it. However, it could not be implemented owing to concerns that it might create a sense of social disharmony. In order to solve the financial problem of NHI, making the related issue public is as important as introducing a for−profit medical corporation. In the US healthcare system, this concept is not necessary as health insurance is not mandated in the country. On the contrary, with the state−owned healthcare system, the UK government employed the pay bed unit available in some of the hospitals.

In the United Kingdom, private insurance covers the medical fee for the occupant of a pay bed, and specialists with a certain level of career can spend some of their working hours to treat the pay−bed patients within a separate medical fee payment system. The pay bed unit exists not only in for−profit hospitals founded by individuals but also in state−owned hospitals, and specialists in the state−owned hospital can also work for the pay beds in their hospital or in any private for−profit hospital for a certain proportion of their working hours. This is to compensate for the limited salary system of doctors in the UK who are quasi−public servants.

The pay bed system is advantageous for both NHI and patients theoretically as the concept will save the spending of NHI and provide patients with a chance to receive a high−quality medical service. However, the public sentiment is against it, claiming that the majority of beds could be neglected because of pay beds that account for only 10−20% of the beds in total. However, we need to discuss this concept once again because the income from 10% of patients can be used to provide a better service for 90% of patients. We need momentum to discuss the necessity of institutional changes that rarely happened in Korea since health insurance was introduced in 1977. The focus of the discussion on health insurance has always been fixed on assuring equity. It is unfortunate that the discussion about pay bed was not developed further despite its potential of killing two birds with one stone.

3. The Necessity of Further Discussion and Policy Direction

The advocates might argue based on the following logic. First, the foreign case studies imply that not many people will use for−profit hospitals. The dissenters assume that the National Health Insurance Act should be amended to introduce a for−profit medical corporation and concern that it would upset the foundation of the NHI system, namely, the mandatory designation system of medical institutions and the mandatory subscription. However, such an amendment requires significant efforts to persuade a group in the National Assembly that is larger than the opposing group, and that is why they are opposing the introduction as they see the amendment is unlikely to happen.

A country with this scale of the economy should be open to every possibility apart from some special cases. To achieve openness in our society, opportunities to meet people's demands and desires should be respected. Koreans have strong demand for equality, so empirical data and research are required to determine whether or not the NHI system should change when we allow the introduction of for−profit hospitals, followed by the discussion on practical matters. In the meantime, the government should be able to assure those who oppose the policy that existing systems, either NHI or health care, will remain solid. The Roh Moo−Hyun administration dealt with expanding and strengthening public health services together when discussing the issue of a for−profit hospital.

Even the most desirable policy will be of no use if it fails to persuade the opposition and is not legislated. Thus, the key point of this issue depends on how to convince the opposition. If the government institutionally guarantees that the NHI system will not be faltered and comes up with a conclusion supported by the empirical verification with specific data, e.g., the gain and loss for each bracket, the opposition should accept the decision. Unfortunately, given the present circumstance within the Ministry of Health and Welfare in relation to the health care and NHI policies, there seems to be no group to drive the agenda in such direction. Even a few scholars who used to be in favor of opening the market no longer speak out. Although the system has been partially mended for the sake of extensive public health and coverage, there is no group to lead a meaningful paradigm shift. Despite the long discussion about public health policies and the marketization and industrialization of the health care industry under the two administrations for the last 10 years, the force to support it has not been matured at all. What we need are a mature movement and supporting groups.

It is true that multiple possibilities need to be considered to meet demand at various levels on a scale similar to the Korean economy. However, foreign cases with various models do not always include everyone. Even though some worry about the polarization, if people with high income are expected to use a greater portion of the medical service, their payment could save some of the NHI spending that could be used to support medical fees for those with lower income; the system can be designed for a fair deal for the low−income bracket. Bracing for the controversy that might be sparked by concerns related to coverage extension, the mandatory designation system, and the mandatory subscription, and the privatization of medical service, the government should develop the discussion by engaging actively in the policy debate with the opposition and promising to reinforce the national policy for the essential public health sector.

The permission of a for−profit medical corporation might not necessarily indicate huge revenue to the Korean healthcare industry. However, it might not cause damage to our healthcare sector as much as the dissenter's claims. The side effect will not be substantial as long as the government keeps consistency in its policy, e.g., maintaining the mandatory designation system and extending the public function in the health insurance as an alternative. As society grows mature, a variety of demands should be respected. Any needs for advanced healthcare service should be considered with open possibilities. Most importantly, collecting empirical data is necessary for mature, balanced discussion.

Section 4

Conflicts of Various Issues Following Separation of Prescribing and Dispensing

1. Progress from 1963 to just before implementing separation of prescribing and dispensing

- **1963:** The principle of separation of prescribing and dispensing (also known as dispensing separation) was stipulated in the revision of the Pharmaceutical Affairs Act, but implementation conditions were sufficient.
- **1965:** As the Addendum of the Pharmaceutical Affairs Act allowed direct dispensing by doctors, the implementation of dispensing separation was practically deferred.
- **1965, 1969:** At the recommendation of the Health and Social Affairs Committee, various committees were formed to promote and implement dispensing separation, but such attempts foundered.
- **1982 to 1985:** As part of the regional medical insurance pilot project, a pilot project for dispensing separation was carried out in Mokpo-si, which ended up being terminated due to the failure to extend the contract in the healthcare and pharmaceutical sectors.
  - First: July, 1982 to April, 1984 Voluntary separation
  - Second: May, 1984 to December, 1984 Forced separation by contract between parties
  - Third: April, 1985 to September, 1985 Voluntary separation
- **1988:** In accordance with the expansion of the National Health Insurance, the "National Healthcare Policy Review Committee" prepared a three-phase plan for implementing dispensing separation.
  - Phase 1: Voluntary dispensing separation induced by insurance reimbursement for pharmaceutical costs (insurance benefits only granted for prescribing and dispensing in accordance with dispensing separation)
  - Phase 2: Enforced dispensing separation for prescription drugs excluding injections
  - Phase 3: Enforced dispensing separation for prescription drugs including injections
- **1989:** As the agreement between doctors and pharmacists was abolished in the legislative process, the pharmacy insurance system was temporarily implemented in July, 1989, until the implementation of dispensing separation, under the purview of stabilizing medical insurance finances by reflecting the medical practices of the people.

- **1993:** In January, 1994, the Pharmaceutical Affairs Act was amended in order to clarify the roles between specialized professions in the wake of the conflict between traditional Korean medicine doctors and pharmacists, and the basic framework for the implementation of dispensing separation was prepared, which was stipulated to be implemented from the data specified by a Presidential decree between July, 1997 to July, 1999.
- **December, 1997:** The "Healthcare Reform Committee," an advisory body of the Prime Minister, suggested a basic model for the phased dispensing separation according to the drug classification method.
  - Phase 1 (1999): Limited prescription drugs such as antibiotics, steroids, and habit-forming drugs
  - Phase 2 (2002): Prescription drugs excluding injections
  - Phase 3 (2005): All prescription drugs
- **May, 1998:** In order to come up with an implementation plan for dispensing separation that suits our situation, the "Council for Separation of Prescribing and Dispensing" was formed with representatives of public interest such as consumer groups and the media as well as experts from the healthcare and pharmaceutical sectors.
- **August 24, 1998:** An agreement on the implementation plan for dispensing separation was achieved at the fourth meeting.

A. Agreement on the implementation plan for by the Council for Separation of Prescribing and Dispensing

The basic principles of dispensing separation agreed in August 1998 were as follows. First, the implementation plan for dispensing separation was pursued in accordance with the current law. Second, dispensing separation was implemented from July 1, 1999. Third, dispensing separation was promoted in a way to minimize the burden and inconvenience to the public on the premise of the participation of professionals in the healthcare and pharmaceutical sectors.

The detailed implementation plan was as follows. First, the pharmaceutical products for which dispensing separation was applied included all prescription drugs excluding injections. Second, mandatory issuance of prescriptions for outpatients was stipulated in the Medical Service Act. However, for a hospital−level or higher healthcare institution that must have a dispensing room under the Medical Service Act. The prescription was issued in a format that did not distinguish between inpatients and outpatients, leaving them to choose between in−hospital and off−hospital dispensing. Third, pharmaceutical products listed in the prescription should be indicated by their generic or brand names. However, if the brand name is written with the indication of "non−substitutable," it can be substituted with a pharmaceutical product that has undergone bioequivalence testing and was announced by the Minister of Health and Welfare. Alternatively, products to other pharmaceutical products may be administered with the consent of the doctor. Nevertheless, in order to address the inconvenience of the public, the Local Council for Separation of Prescribing and Dispensing notified the pharmacies of the list of medications under the brand names allowed for administration.

Related recommendations included taking measures to minimize pharmaceutical product price margins. These include transactions, supplementing insurance fee systems in which outpatient prescription issuance was more advantageous compared to in−hospital. Preparing institutional improvement plans to establish the healthcare delivery system as soon as possible, and prevention from being distorted by the dispensing separation.

Nevertheless, between November and December 1998, the Korean Medical Association, the Korean Hospital Association, and the Korean Pharmaceutical Association each filed a petition to delay the implementation of the dispensing separation in the National Assembly. This was due to members' objections to the agreement reached in the fourth meeting of the Council for Separation of Prescribing and Dispensing on August 24, 1998. On February 18, 1999, the National Congress for New Politics decided that it was impossible to promote dispensing separation without a new agreement between the healthcare and pharmaceutical organizations on the implementation plan. As an agreement was not reached despite the arbitration attempt with a mediation at the policy committee level, it was decided to proceed according to the government plan (the plan of the Council for Separation of Prescribing and Dispensing).

B. Plan for separation and implementation of prescribing and dispensing

On March 2 1993, the Korean Medical Association and the Korean Pharmaceutical Association, under the joint name, postponed the implementation by one year to prepare dispensing separation at healthcare institutions and pharmacies, and agreed to develop a new dispensing separation model in collaboration with civic and consumer groups. In case of failure, they agreed to proceed according to the government's plan.

On March 31 1999, the National Assembly accepted the recommendation of the Korean Medical Association and the Korean Pharmaceutical Association and revised the Pharmaceutical Affairs Act. This led to delayed implementation of dispensing separation by one year to July 1 2000 (Sang—young Lee, 2008)[85].

Based on the recommendation of the Korean Medical Association and the Korean Pharmaceutical Association, on March 30, 1999. The "Citizens Countermeasure Committee for Dispensing Separation," was formed including the Citizens' Coalition for Economic Justice, People's Solidarity for Participatory Democracy, Green Consumer Network in Korea, Consumers Union of Korea, and YMCA. They proposed a plan to implement dispensing separation agreed upon by representatives of the healthcare and pharmaceutical sectors after six open discussions and public hearings on May 10, 1999. The plan for dispensing separation by the Citizens Countermeasure Committee was as follow.

---

85) Sang—young Lee, A Study for Comprehensive Evaluation of Dispensing Separation and System Improvement Planning, Korea Institute for Health and Social Affairs, 2008.

- **Institutions**
: Outpatient dispensing rooms at healthcare institutions are closed to make off-hospital dispensing mandatory for outpatients in all healthcare institutions (including community health centers and their branch offices).
- **Pharmaceutical products**
: Prescription drugs, including injections (those that require safety for transport and storage, anticancer drugs, and injections for testing, surgery, and treatment may be excluded according to the decision of the Central Pharmaceutical Affairs Council)
- **Prescription issuance method**
: Pharmaceutical products are prescribed by brand name or generic name. With prescriptions under the brand name, alternative preparations are permitted with the pharmaceutical products of the same ingredient, content, and formulation, which the patients need to be informed beforehand and the doctor notified later.
- **Ensuring therapeutic equivalence**
: All pharmaceutical products are re-evaluated prior to dispensing separation to ensure their therapeutic equivalence, and non-efficacious drugs removed.
- **Classification, labeling, and storage of pharmaceutical products**
: Classification of prescription and over-the-counter drugs is based on the National Assembly adjustment plan, but items that need re-examination are identified by the Central Pharmaceutical Affairs Council after objective research were by the end of March, 2000 (full re-classification every three years). Separate labels are placed on the packaging of prescription and over-the-counter drugs, and stored separately, and an identification symbol printed on each medicine.
- **Administration of over-the-counter drugs**
: Sale of over-the-counter drugs with their packaging opened by pharmacists is prohibited (however, PTP or foil labeled with ingredient names, contents and manufacturer is considered as packaging).
- **Improvement of related systems**
: For preparing and checking the implementation of dispensing separation, the measures such as the formation of the Committee on Separation of Prescribing and Dispensing, the implementation of the healthcare delivery system and the regular family doctor/pharmacist system until dispensing separation, the introduction of Good Pharmacy Practice (GPP) Standards, night-time care at community health centers, the prohibition of collusion between healthcare institutions and pharmacies, and the preparation of the Act on Remedies for Injuries from Medical Malpractice and Mediation of Medical Disputes.

In June 1999, based on the agreement and suggestion of the Korean Medical Association and the Korean Pharmaceutical Association, the "Executive Committee on Separation of Prescribing and Dispensing" was formed with healthcare and pharmaceutical—related groups, civic and consumer groups, and the media. Through 11 sectional meetings and two general meetings, various recommendations were reviewed and detailed implementation plans to minimize inconvenience to the public were confirmed (September 17, 1999), and the "Pharmaceutical Affairs Act" was revised based on the plan suggested by the Executive Committee on Separation of Prescribing and Dispensing (January 12, 2000)[86].

---

86) History and Implementation of Dispensing Separation — Naver Blog. [m.blog.naver.com]

2. Background for separation of prescribing and dispensing and the financial problem of National Health Insurance

A. Response of the Council for Separation of Prescribing and Dispensing and civic groups

In 1998, the government, which was not very active in promoting dispensing separation, formed the Council for Separation of Prescribing and Dispensing (hereinafter referred to as the "Dispensing Separation Council") to prepare a plan for dispensing separation. At that time, the Dispensing Separation Council's plan allowed in−hospital dispensing facilities in hospitals and allowed in−hospital dispensing and injections for outpatients with many exceptions allowed. It was a relaxed form, which was closer to function separation rather than dispensing separation, allowing pharmacists to prepare substitutes and alternatives without the consent of doctors.

Dispensing separation began with the conflict between traditional Korean medicine doctors and pharmacists, and the government led by President Dae−Jung Kim implemented it as one of the 100 reform tasks. While the government came up with a relaxed plan by the Dispensing Separation Council, it was kept rejected due to opposition from interested parties. Nevertheless, as the civic groups came into the scene for arbitration, a strict plan was suggested. The government predicted that the plan suggested by the civic groups would not be accepted as even the relaxed plan suggested by the government had been rejected.

However, the political situation at the time happened to empower the civic groups. The public had little confidence in the government, as they had just escaped from the control of the previous authoritarian government. The emergence of new political reformers as well as the rise of civic groups led to the acceptance of the plan.

B. Implementation of drug price reduction and introduction of actual transaction pricing system

The Citizens' Coalition for Economic Justice was at the center of the civic groups. Councilor Yong−ik Kim of the Citizens' Coalition for Economic Justice ultimately aimed at forbidding rebates associated with drugs through dispensing separation. Such an opinion was published in the Joseon Ilbo as an expert contribution, followed by a lot of backlash from the healthcare sector. In addition, he insisted that the price of drugs needed to be reduced. At that time, drug pricing was regulated by the official pricing system. Regarding drug price reduction, the Ministry of Health and Welfare tried to reduce drug prices by more than 30% by conducting actual transaction inspections with civic groups.

There had been many contributing factors, but it can be said that the drug price was the main reason for the sharp change in the dispensing separation situation. As there would be inevitable differences occurring in the process of distributing powers in any form of authority surrounding dispensing separation, it was necessary to minimize the interests associated with drugs. Moreover, it was necessary to minimize the unfair profits for alleviating conflicts in the process of distributing powers in association with drugs, thereby eliminating an undesirable social phenomenon.

As such, the plan for dispensing separation was created by the civic groups as the center. Nevertheless, not all motives in the background of dispensing separation were pure. Under the official pricing system, the drug price margin was officially allowed. However, there was opposing pressure from multinational pharmaceutical companies against the drug price margins. Multinational pharmaceutical companies have consistently insisted on the introduction of the real transaction pricing system and transparency in the operation of the system. Under such circumstances, the actual transaction pricing system was implemented. As a result of investigating the official prices and actual transaction prices, there was about a 29% difference. Such a difference allowed the doctors to receive rebates.

The actual transaction prices were reported, and the drug prices were reduced by 30.7%, which was compensated by the medical fee. As the actual transaction pricing system was implemented in October 1999, the drug price was decreased and the medical fee was increased on November 15, 1999. In November, doctors gathered at the Jangchung Gymnasium to protest against the drug price reduction and to hold a rally and strike against dispensing separation.

C. Increase in medical fee in the National Health Insurance system and financial problems

At that time, Professor Woo−Jin Jung at the Graduate School of Public Health, Yonsei University, who was a researcher at the Korea Institute for Health and Social Affairs, reported that dispensing separation would cost a lot of money. The Health Insurance Bureau of the Ministry of Health and Welfare opposed the promotion of dispensing separation on the grounds that it would cost more based on the report. At that time, the Ministry of Health and Welfare held an expert meeting to review the first prescription dispensing fee while the Director of National Health Insurance Yoon−gu Kang, and the Secretary Yong−jin Eom were in service at the Ministry of Health and Welfare. At that time, representatives from academia, healthcare and pharmaceutical sectors, civic groups gathered.in order to implement dispensing separation, it was necessary to pay doctors the prescription fee and pharmacists the dispensing fee, which would cost more money. Dr. Woo−jin Jung of the Korea Institute for Health and Social Affairs was asked to give a presentation to address this issue. Therefore, Dr. Woo−jin Jung presented that it would cost additional KRW 3 trillion to finance dispensing separation. At the meeting that day, there was a heated discussion with the participants as to whether the Ministry of Health and Welfare was intentionally trying to stop dispensing separation. The atmosphere in the conference room was very intense.

However, such a report would make it politically difficult to promote dispensing separation. The Healthcare Policy Bureau, which was in charge of promoting dispensing separation in the Ministry of Health and Welfare, had presented a report by Professor Bong−min Yang at Graduate School of Public Health, Seoul National University, that the implementation of dispensing separation would greatly reduce the medical expenses of the public to the President, and the President ordered to promote the division of labor based on that report.

It was declared to reduce the public medical expenses; nevertheless, regardless of the cause, the medical fee was raised five times, causing a huge burden on the finances. Doctors were dissatisfied, pharmacists were dissatisfied, and the people were satisfied due to the inconvenience of having to visit a separate pharmacy to receive medication after obtaining the prescription from the hospital. To make matters worse, the finances of the National Health Insurance suffered. Later, it was also said that President Dae−jung Kim told his staff that he was deceived by a false report that dispensing separation would reduce medical expenses when he decided to promote dispensing separation.

As doctors rallied and went on strike on the reform task that the president was interested in, the government became very impatient. As a result, Yun−bae Kim, who was the Senior Secretary to the President for Social Welfare at the time, and his disciple, Secretary Se−hee Cho, had a meeting with Jae−jeong Kim, the Chairman of the Korean Medical Association, in an attempt to solve the issues associated with dispensing separation by themselves, practically excluding the Health and Welfare Planning Office and the Ministry of Health and Welfare. The Ministry of Health and Welfare was excluded from the scene. At first, Chairman Jae−jeong Kim said they would stop protesting in return for an increase in the medical fee even though they were not protesting for the medical fee. Once such a demand was accommodated, other professional groups started making requests. Residents, the Medical Professors Association of Korea, research lecturers, and private practitioners demanded an increase in the medical fee. The negotiations and medical fee increases took place five times, which should have been completed at once.

If the Ministry of Health and Welfare was involved in the negotiation based on its authority and responsibility, there may have been no such result as having to increase the medical fee five times. Due to the direct intervention of the Senior Secretary to the President, the responsibility fell on the President, thereby pulling the noose around the neck of the administration (In the end, the medical fee was properly raised again, and it was resolved in a meeting when Hoi−chang Lee was the leader of the opposition party).

From a policy standpoint, it can be analyzed in various ways. At the end of the day, for a policy to change, the outcome should be greater than the input. It must far outweigh all the social costs required for the change. That is a very essential part, and a change in policy results in a change in the distribution of power. Those who have something to lose are likely to resist. As for dispensing separation, both doctors and pharmacists felt they had something to lose and opposed it. Although the ultimate benefits such as ensuring the right to health from dispensing separation would affect the people, the long−term and microscopic effect on the right to health, which was divided and distributed to all people, was not truly felt by each individual. In a situation with enormous resistance from both doctors and pharmacists, no party except civic groups could speak out with a cause. The implementation of this had been delayed due to the difficulties to begin with.

It was a major event that a policy that could put an excessive financial burden on people at once was introduced in this way. In hindsight, all available means were mobilized as much as possible to bring the healthcare and pharmaceutical sectors into the system of dispensing separation. Raising the medical fee five times was unimaginable. However, it was not that the impact of the policy was not known before it was introduced. The president at that time, who had no choice but to push the system despite the obvious difficulties, must have experienced a great anguish.

Upon raising the medical fee on September 1, 2000, the Health Insurance Bureau also opposed it. The Director of the Health Insurance Bureau did not approve the increase in the medical fee. Based on the agreement between the government and the healthcare and pharmaceutical sectors, the tasks associated with the medical fee were carried out at a hotel in Gwacheon. On September 1, 2000, the National Health Insurance Act was amended. At that time, the amended law stated to increase the medical fee based on a contract, which was neglected by the Minister of Health and Welfare who ordered the medical fee to be raised. As the Minister of Health and Welfare took the post, he insisted that the medical fee was lower than the cost. Due to the unfair increase in the medical fee, the health insurance bureau drafted a proposal on September 1, and was approved. Nonetheless, the medical fee was increased on September 1, which was pointed out by the civic groups as a problem. As the National Health Insurance Act was amended on July 1, 2000, the National Health Insurance Act was passed to allow adjusting the medical cost based on a contract, but the Ministry of Health and Welfare peremptorily decided to raise the medical fee.

From the standpoint of subscribers, the important aim of introducing the medical fee contract system was to increase the medical cost considering the opinions of subscriber groups as much as possible, not by a unilateral announcement from the Minister. As the medical fee kept increasing despite the opposition of the National Health Insurance, such a provision was prepared as a legal safety pin. Meanwhile, from the standpoint of the Ministry of Health and Welfare, it was intended to provide a way out of the interference of the Ministry of Economy and Finance within the government in raising the medical fee. In other words, prior to a notification, the medical fee had to be negotiated with the Ministry of Economy and Finance each time, and it was subject to the inflation rate each time. In the medical fee contract system, the Ministry of Economy and Finance became one of the many parties involved in the contract, with reduced influence over the matter. Since other countries had already been implementing a system for medical fee contracts based on agreement, there was a discussion about using this system in South Korea as well. Therefore, the Council of Medical Care Benefit Organizations was established, and the National Health Insurance Act was enacted to designate the representatives of the National Health Insurance Corporation and the Council of Medical Care Benefit Organizations as parties in the contract.

Prior to the enactment of the National Health Insurance Act, the Ministry of Economy and Finance, the department in charge of prices and budgets, took the lead in the decision−making process for increasing the medical fee in a superior position than the Ministry of Health and Welfare, and the department in charge of health insurance. As the provision on the medical fee contract system was included in the law, the status of the Ministry of Economy and Finance was reduced to one of the parties involved in the contract. As the authority of the Ministry of Health and Welfare, the Health Insurance Corporation, and the subscribers were relatively strengthened, the authority that had been concentrated in the Ministry of Economy and Finance was distributed.

At that time, in the process of prior consultation with the Ministry of Economy and Finance for increasing the medical fee on September 1, the director at the Ministry of Economy and Finance opposed the increase in the medical fee and marked it with a "No." In addition to the "No," he added an X mark with a comment saying, "It is against the law." Later, the stance was changed. Under such circumstances, the civic groups filed a lawsuit with the Constitutional Court on September 1, claiming that the increase in the medical fee was a violation of the law. The Constitutional Court dismissed it with five votes in favor of and four against the decision on unconstitutionality. When six or more votes were in favor of the decision on unconstitutionality, such an increase in the medical fee would have been found to be unconstitutional, thereby nullifying the increase in the medical fee. However, four of the judges sided with the government.

Even after dispensing separation, the government and the healthcare and pharmaceutical sectors continued to hold legislative and contract meetings. They tried to describe the contents and reflect them to a considerable extent in the amendment of the law. The finances that had been broken for a short period of time with the introduction of dispensing separation was recovered.

What was not realized until the end was the implementation of the reference pricing system. The former Minister Tae−bok Lee contributed to the failure to implement the reference pricing system. For the implementation of the reference pricing system, the government suggested a plan to set the reference price at 150% of the average price by grouping the drugs based on their efficacy, and this alone could save a lot of money. Former Minister Tae−bok Lee who was serving as the Senior Secretary to the President for Social Welfare insisted on setting the reference price at 50% of the average price. The Division of Health Insurance Benefits of the Ministry of Health and Welfare was against the opinion based on the reason that while only the civic groups agreed to the reference pricing system in the absence of scientific grounds for therapeutic equivalence, excessive burden on the patient would make the civic groups turn their back on the policy, thereby making it impossible to implement the system. At that time, according to the plan by the Ministry of Health and Welfare, the estimated amount of financial savings was about KRW 300 billion, and the amount was estimated to double based on the calculation of Senior Secretary Tae−bok Lee. He wanted to use the additional savings for the welfare of the elderly. However, as the savings of the National Health Insurance finances were not a part of the general budget, they could not be directly used as a budget for the welfare of the elderly.

The Chief of the Division of Health Insurance Benefits remarked that there were no scientific grounds despite causing a great burden on the patients, and that the policy would fail. While the amount of savings was calculated to increase, there would be no savings in the end as the policy was destined to fail. Due to such controversies, the reference pricing system ended up not being implemented. What was difficult in the calculations to prepare for the implementation of the system was that the Health Insurance Review and Assessment Service did not have a database at the time, and each calculation had to be performed one by one through re−programing with a magnetic tape during the night time after work.

Another policy that was not properly implemented was related to therapeutic equivalence. When determining the items for drug substitution, only the pharmaceutical products with therapeutic equivalence were recognized as substitutes. There would be no problem in association with efficacy equivalence if it was ensured by thorough clinical trials. Nevertheless, due to the arousal of controversies over drug substitution, doctors started to question therapeutic equivalence to back up their argument against drug substitution. Doctors pointed out that the clinical trials were not being conducted properly in South Korea. Therefore, the therapeutic equivalence tests had to be conducted again, while there were not enough clinical trial institutions to handle the sudden surge of items for testing. At that time, if the price of the original pharmaceutical product was 100, that of the first generic product was 80, and the second 60, dropping by 20%. The testing of therapeutic equivalence started at the same time, but it was advantageous to finish the testing sooner as the drug was more likely to be highly priced. The therapeutic equivalence testing was carried out by force, and the testing institutions were not mature enough. The therapeutic equivalence was falsely reported to the Food and Drug Administration, which led to subsequent problems.

Since the solid setup upon the promotion of dispensing separation, there has never been a single change in the designation of prescription and over−the−counter drugs unlike the examples in developed countries. It may have been because such a decision was made as a result of a great struggle. The first change to the initial setup was probably the decision made by the administration led by President Myung−bak Lee to allow the sales of pharmaceutical products at supermarkets.

3. Implementation and supplementation of separation of prescribing and dispensing

A. Supplementation after implementation

In November 1999, when the implementation plan for dispensing separation was being finalized, the Ministry of Health and Welfare improved the medical insurance drug pricing system for smooth implementation of dispensing separation. This unexpectedly triggered the healthcare sector to express their ongoing dissatisfaction with the health insurance program as well as the healthcare system. The drug pricing system for medical insurance was changed from the existing "official price reimbursement method" to the "actual price reimbursement method." The healthcare sector players were dissatisfied that the drug price margin, which had been granted, disappeared overnight due to dispensing separation. Although the Ministry of Health and Welfare announced a plan to compensate for the reduced drug costs through the new drug pricing system by increasing the medical fee for doctors. However, the government and the healthcare sector did not have enough trust to overcome dissatisfaction. On November 30 1999, the healthcare sector including the Korean Medical Association held a large−scale rally at Jangchung Gymnasium in Seoul to discredit Chairman Seong−hee Yoo of the Korean Medical Association. He had signed the agreement on May 10 and approved the "Committee for the Struggle for Doctors' Rights", a key component to the struggle against dispensing separation. In the end, the healthcare sector enforced closures of medical institutions nationwide in June, February and April of 2000, and those leading the protest including the Chairman of the Korean Medical Association and Chairman of the Committee for the Struggle for Doctors' Rights, were arrested. These eventually led the residents and professors at university hospitals join the protest, resulting in failure of the healthcare system[87].

---

87) Ministry of Health and Welfare, "70 Years of Health and Welfare" Volume 2 Healthcare Edition, 2016.

To resolve the chaos caused by the overall closure in the healthcare sector, in June, President Dae—jung Kim and the opposition party leader, Hoi—chang Lee, held a joint summit. The collective happening in the healthcare sector made the people become critical toward dispensing separation, causing a political burden. This was a major crisis in the implementation of dispensing separation. Nevertheless, the government maintained a firm stance on dispensing separation, leading to a chain of implementations. In the summit, the opposition party leader, Hoi—chang Lee agreed with the healthcare sector in the stance of "implementation after supplementation."

However, President Dae—jung Kim did not accept this, and decided to make necessary amendments to the "Pharmaceutical Affairs Act" while carrying out dispensing separation. As it was decided to make an amendment to the "Pharmaceutical Affairs Act" in the provisional session of the National Assembly in July because of the summit between the ruling—party and opposition leaders. The National Assembly Health and Welfare Committee's Subcommittee on Separation of Prescribing and Dispensing decided to limit the scope of the amendment to the sale of over—the—counter drugs' out of their packaging and drug substitution. The government agreed to draft an agreement with the healthcare, pharmaceutical, and civil groups by July 1 and submit it to the National Assembly. The Ministry of Health and Welfare closely consulted on this issue on June 29 and 30 with the Korean Medical Association, the Korean Hospital Association, the Korean Pharmaceutical Association, and the civic groups participating in the Citizens Countermeasure Committee. The healthcare and pharmaceutical groups refrained from giving an opinion as they either had submitted a petition for amendment to the "Pharmaceutical Affairs Act" or were planning to submit a petition. In the end, the National Assembly incorporated the opinions from the Korean Medical Association, the Korean Pharmaceutical Association, and the civic groups, and decided to draft and submit a final agreement by July 7. The Ministry of Health and Welfare prepared a draft agreement after all—night negotiations with the Korean Medical Association and the Korean Pharmaceutical Association "to prescribe and dispense medicines within the scope of medicines stipulated by the regional Cooperation Council for Dispensing Separation, and to forbid the sale of over—the—counter medicines with the packaging open by pharmacists."

However, due to the refusal to accept some of the contents of the agreement by the Committee for the Struggle for Doctors' Rights, a resolution could not be reached. The Ministry of Health and Welfare continued consulting with the healthcare, pharmaceutical and civic groups even after reporting its progress to the National Assembly on July 10. Although no complete consensus was reached, the opinions on the amendment to the "Pharmaceutical Affairs Act" were organized focusing on the contents to generally reflect the views of each group, on July 13, 2000.

Opinions gathered through twists and turns were reflected in the amendment to the "Pharmaceutical Affairs Act" on August 5,2000, in the form of legislation. In respect of the preparations at the pharmacies, healthcare institutions, the adaptation of the people to the system, and publicity, dispending separation was implemented from August 1 after one—month pilot from July 1, 2000.

B. Supplementation of the policy for the separation of prescribing and dispensing

The Ministry of Health and Welfare established a task force for dispensing separation to carry out various public relations campaigns in collaboration with the local government. This was because even after dispensing separation was implemented after the pilot, there were many complaints from patients. Also, the active participation of the healthcare sector could not be gotten, and the pharmacies also had difficulties in procuring prescription drugs. Eventually, the task force for dispensing separation was overwhelmed with phone calls from dissatisfied patients.

The healthcare sector workers went on a strike on October 5, 2000, demanding the proper implementation of the dispensing separation and re−amendment to the Pharmaceutical Affairs Act. Outpatient treatment at tertiary hospitals, university hospitals, local clinics and small to medium−sized hospitals were completely closed.

In the early stages of implementing dispensing separation, people's inconvenience was associated with unfamiliar new systems and the frequent industrial actions of the healthcare sector workers were impossible to overcome even though the Ministry of Health and Welfare kept open communication with the healthcare and pharmaceutical sectors. Through the 26 sessions of "the dialog between the government and the healthcare sector" from September 26, 2000, as well as six sessions of "the dialog between the government and the pharmaceutical sector" from October 31, a comprehensive agreement on the supplementation of dispensing separation was reached on November 11, 2000. The agreement of the government with the healthcare and pharmaceutical sectors was submitted to the National Assembly as a legislative proposal after a joint signing ceremony by the Chairman of the Korean Medical Association (Jae−jeong Kim), the Chairman of the Korean Pharmaceutical Association (Hee−joong Kim), and the Minister of Health and Welfare (Seon−jeong Choi)− that formed a council. This event took place at the office of the Chairman of the National Assembly Health and Welfare Committee on December 11, 2000.

The council of the government with the healthcare and pharmaceutical sectors resolved conflicts that had occurred in the process of promoting dispensing separation and promised to make efforts based on mutual trust and cooperation between the government and the healthcare and pharmaceutical sectors. The agreed systematic improvements related to dispensing separation were summarized as follows[88].

---

88) Unsolved problem for 20 years of dispensing separation. The disappearance of the "promise to submit the list of prescription" − Hit News. [www.hitnews.co.kr]

〈Results of the council meeting between the government and the healthcare and pharmaceutical sectors regarding the separation of prescribing and dispensing〉

First, the healthcare and pharmaceutical sectors as well as the government sincerely apologize for causing excessive inconvenience and suffering to the public due to the lack of cooperation in the introduction and implementation of dispensing separation.

The government and the healthcare and pharmaceutical sectors have reached a consensus that dispensing separation was a system necessary to advance the healthcare system, and needs to be implemented.

In addition, we agreed inconvenience inevitably occurred in the early stage of implementation of the new dispensing separation. We are hopeful this will be resolved through trust and cooperation of the healthcare and pharmaceutical sectors.

In the future, based on mutual trust and cooperation built through dialogue among the government, the healthcare and pharmaceutical sectors, we solemnly pledge to make efforts at early settlement of dispensing separation through active participation and ensure safe and convenient prescription and dispensing.

1. The healthcare sector shall:
· Submit the local prescription drug list with an adequate number of items for, and select the drugs with excellent quality and reasonable price as much as possible.
· Mark "non-substitutable" only when it is necessary according to strict standards.
· Cooperate when pharmacists request for drug substitution under unavoidable circumstances.
· Reduce the rate of prescription of injections and actively educate patients to use oral medications.
2. The pharmaceutical sector shall:
· Provide a thorough instruction on drug administration.
· Refer patients suspected of having certain diseases to a doctor.
· Respect the opinions of doctors in selecting the prescription from drug list.
· Make sure to procure the pharmaceutical products on the local prescription drug list.
· Curtail the case of dispensing without prescription.
3. The healthcare and pharmaceutical sectors shall:
· Strive to improve the quality of prescribing and dispensing through mutual exchange of opinions and education.
· Cooperate with each other for the improvement and development of the healthcare and pharmaceutical system.
· Monitor and eradicate collusion between healthcare institutions and pharmacies.
· Carry out reform work to overcome any internal negative factors.
4. The government shall
: Provide institutional support to improve the health of the people through development of the healthcare and pharmaceutical sectors.

Dispensing separation is formed by combining various systems such as classification of prescription and over－the－counter drugs, methods of prescribing and dispensing, manufacturing, import approval and review standards, and drug supply such as distribution and sales. Therefore, there are many difficulties in assessing dispensing separation because the effects of the dispensing separation are widespread and manifest over a long period of time. Through dispensing separation, the conventional practice of random formulation by pharmacists was prevented, and the disclosure of prescription rooted out the "secret prescription" which lacked scientific grounds. The perspectives on the pharmaceutical market have changed, and the domestic pharmaceutical industry and distribution system have been completely reorganized. The quality of domestic medicines was improved through bioequivalence testing. Furthermore, by establishing a drug safety management system, advanced safety policies such as drug utilization review (DUR), drug prescribing and dispensing support service could be implemented.

Section 5

Traditional Korean Medicine Policy and Conflict between Traditional Korean Medicine Doctors and Pharmacists

1. Introduction and Progress of Traditional Korean Medicine Policy

The License System for oriental medical doctors was officially introduced in 1951, and developed since the promotion of the Policy that resolved the conflict between oriental medical doctors and pharmacists in 1993. In June 1993, a department in charge of traditional Korean medicine was established within the Ministry of Health and Social Affairs with a designated officer. This expanded and reorganized the traditional Korean medicine policy. Two officers, each in charge of traditional Korean medicine service and promotion, were designated to develop the Office. Starting with the establishment of the Herbal Medicine Division at the Ministry of Food and Drug Safety in 1998, the Herbal Medicine Management and Evaluation Teams were established in 2006. These were then reorganized into the Herbal Medicine Policy and the Traditional Korean Medicine Industry Divisions in February, 2008 and laid a foundation for carrying out policies related to the medicine industry[89].

In 1994, the government made investment following the establishment of the department through the creation of the Korea Research Institute of Oriental Medicine—a research institute for traditional Korean medicine. In 1998, the Traditional Korean Medicine Technology Development Project, "2010 Project (1998 to 2007)," was executed, and further advances made through the enactment of the "Oriental Medicine Promotion Act" in 2003; the establishment of the comprehensive plan for the "First Five—year Development of Traditional Korean Medicine (2006 to 2010)" in 2005; the installation of the "Graduate School of Oriental Medicine at Busan University" in 2008; the establishment of the comprehensive plan for the "Second Five—year Development of Traditional Korean Medicine (2011 to 2015)" in 2010; and the establishment of the comprehensive plan for the "Third Five—year Development of Traditional Korean Medicine (2016 to 2020)" (Jong—Yeol Kim, 2016)[90].

---

89) Hye—jeong Lee, Pump Primer for Fostering the Traditional Korean Medicine Industry. Report of Korean Medicine Policy, Vol.1 No.1 2016.

90) Jong—Yeol Kim (2016). Current Status of Traditional Korean Medicine Industry and Direction of Policies.

The herbal pharmacist system has been developed since the conflicts over the dispensing of herbal medicines in 1993, through the establishment of the Korea Institute of Oriental Medicine in 1994, the introduction of the herbal pharmacist system in 1996, the introduction of the specialist system in 2000, and the introduction of the public health doctor system in 2002. In the field of public healthcare, a traditional Korean medicine doctor was first deployed to (a branch office of) a community health centers in a rural area to carry out health projects and provide oriental medicine treatment in 1998. In 2001, the pilot project of the public health promotion programs in traditional Korean medicine was conducted. In 2002, the regional health project in traditional Korean medicine was promoted in connection with existing projects, and the evaluation of the medicine industry was conducted in 2003. Community centers were selected to provide traditional Korean medicine and named the hub. The number of hub community health centers were expanded to 23 in 2005 with eight programs introduced, and 85 designated in 2012 to carry out various public health promotion programs. In 2013, the public health promotion programs were implemented by integrating the local communities, and the Public Evaluation Group for Traditional Korean Medicine integrated in 2014 into the Korea Health Promotion Institute. As a result, the public health promotion programs in traditional Korean medicine were both mandatory and selective projects from 2005 to 2012. From 2013 to 2014, the priority and selective projects were based on the category of disease. After 2015, the health promotion programs in traditional Korean medicine were conducted throughout the life cycle.

Meanwhile, after the introduction of the herbal medicine standardization system in 1997, the use of standardized products became mandatory in 2007, and the real—name herbal medicine distribution system was implemented in 2005. In addition, the herbal medicine supply and demand control system has been in operation since 1998 to revitalize the production of Korean herbal medicines.

In 2003, the "Oriental Medicine Promotion Act" was enacted to prepare the legal grounds for the development of traditional Korean medicine. Based on this, the "First Comprehensive Plan for the Development of Traditional Korean Medicine (2006 to 2010)" was developed and implemented in 2006, and the "Second (2011 to 2015)" in 2011.

In August 1975, the government decided on the establishment of the herbal medicine department at a Cabinet meeting and promulgated the Ministry of Health and Social Affairs decree. The main intent of this amended decree was, "to establish Divisions 1, 2, and 3 in the Healthcare Policy Bureau. The Division 3 was responsible for reorganization of systems and laws in the field of oriental medicine, R&D and awareness projects, supply—demand planning and training of traditional Korean medicine officials, guidance and supervision of medicine groups as well as practitioners and acupuncturists, and the development of products and research on medical devices for traditional Korean medicine." In March 1977, tasks such as dental affairs, oral health, nursing, and healthcare equipment were added to the responsibilities of Healthcare Policy Division 3. In November 1981, the law was amended through a Presidential decree to close Healthcare Policy Department 3, and the tasks associated with traditional Korean medicine were transferred to the Healthcare System Division of the Healthcare Policy Bureau. This reduced the category, under "R&D of oriental medicine."

The medical insurance coverage for traditional Korean medicine started in February 1987 after a pilot project from December 1984 to November 1986. After the implementation of the medical protection system in 1979, the benefits of traditional Korean medicine protection for recipients of the livelihood program started on January 1 1993, seven years later. Accordingly, medical protection was also applied to traditional Korean medicine protection in March 1993. These included the contents of the review of the Medical Insurance Association and to the revision of the enforcement decree for the implementation of traditional Korean medicine protection for medical protection recipients. In 1993, traditional Korean medicine protection was provided to medical protection recipients, eliminating the difference in the coverage of medical insurance for western medicine. On November 19 1992, the Minister of Health and Social Affairs gave a legislative notice of amendment to the Enforcement Decree of the "Medical Insurance Act" to relieve the burden of medical expenses for low–income citizens. The main content of the amendment was to allow traditional Korean medicine clinics and hospitals to be designated as medical protection institutions. In addition, it contained the reviews on administrative work procedures for practical application of the traditional Korean medicine protection such as the healthcare institution bill statement form for inpatient and outpatient treatments at traditional Korean medicine hospital, the outpatient treatment at healthcare institution, and the medical billing system. It was an attempt to review the laws for implementation of the traditional Korean medicine protection project for medical protection recipients, showing the desire of the government for the active involvement in the medical protection project.

Following the conflict between traditional Korean medicine doctors and pharmacists, the department in charge of traditional Korean medicine was reinstalled. In June 1993, the traditional Korean medicine office was newly designated as a temporary organization in the Healthcare Policy Bureau (Ministry of Health and Social Affairs decree), and changed to a regular organization in July, 1995. In November 1996, the Traditional Korean and Herbal Medicine Policy Officer was established for the first time as an independent bureau–level organization in charge of traditional Korean medicine.

The change of name to the Traditional Korean and Herbal Medicine Policy Officer incorporated traditional Korean medicine–based healthcare and herbal medicine as the means of treatment. This clarified the meaning as well as the aim upon establishing or promoting the policy.

In January 2003, the Ministry of Health and Welfare announced a legislative notice of the Enforcement Decree of the Food Sanitation Act, for administrative monitoring of imported herbal medicines. In January 2004, the Korea Food and Drug Administration formed the Promotion Group of R&D for New Drugs Made of Natural Product as an advisory body, and the National Herbal Medicine Quality Science Research Group was launched in May 2005. In August 2006, the Korean Food and Drug Administration established the Herbal Medicine Management Team and the Herbal Medicine Evaluation Team. In April 2009, the Herbal Medicine Evaluation Department of the Herbal Medicine Quality Division merged into the Herbal Medicine Policy Division, and the Herbal Medicine Standards Division and the Herbal Medicine Evaluation Team of the Herbal Medicine Division were merged into the Herbal Medicine Division. As the Korean Food and Drug Administration was promoted to the Ministry of Food and Drug Safety and transferred to the Prime Minister's Office in 2013, the current affairs related to herbal medicine are being handled by the Herbal Medicine Policy Division of the Biopharmaceuticals and Herbal

Medicine Bureau[91]).

In January 1991, the National Medical Center opened the Traditional Korean Medicine Department with 46 beds and six outpatient clinics (Traditional Korean Medicine, Acupuncture, and Herbal Therapy). Since its relaunch in April 2010, the National Medical Center has been composed of and operated with three departments: Traditional Korean Internal Medicine, Traditional Korean Neuropsychiatry, and Acupuncture.

Meanwhile, in the process of resolving the first conflict between traditional Korean medicine doctors triggered by the amendment to the Enforcement Rules of the Pharmaceutical Affairs Act in March 1993, the government announced the promotion of a five—point policy for the development of traditional Korean medicine, including the establishment of a national institute of traditional Korean medicine. Accordingly, the Korea Research Institute of Oriental Medicine Act was enacted in March 1994. In August 1994, the Korea Research Institute of Oriental Medicine started research activities with the official approval. In August 1996, the Ministry of Health and Welfare announced that the Korea Research Institute of Oriental Medicine would be expanded and reorganized into the Korea Institute of Oriental Medicine in the development plan for fostering traditional Korean medicine. In July 1997, the "Korean Institute of Oriental Medicine Act" was amended and the Korea Research Institute of Oriental Medicine was promoted to the Korea Institute of Oriental Medicine.

2. Background and progress of conflict between traditional Korean medicine doctors and pharmacists

A. Background of conflict between traditional Korean medicine doctors and pharmacists

The "conflict between traditional Korean medicine doctors and pharmacists," which heated up the South Korean society in 1993, was triggered by the amendment to the Enforcement Rules of the Pharmaceutical Affairs Act by the Ministry of Health and Social Affairs. This was due to the provision to "keep medicine cabinets other than traditional herbal medicine cabinets in pharmacies and keep them clean," commonly known as the "traditional herbal medicine cabinet" provision was deleted in March of the same year. Nevertheless, behind the scenes, there had been a deep—rooted conflict between interest groups over "herbal medicine" for a long time.

First of all, detailed story of the "traditional herbal medicine cabinet" provision to be included in the Enforcement Decree of the Pharmaceutical Affairs Act started with the National Assembly, receiving a petition from the Korean Medical Association that urged the government to ban the arbitrary dispensing of herbal medicines and the performance of traditional Korean medicine therapy by pharmacists. This was a supplementary resolution related to the amendment to the Enforcement Rules of the Pharmaceutical Affairs Act in 1975. In December 1976, Young—rok Park and 55 other members of the New Democratic Party at the time proposed a draft of the amendment

---

91) 10 Major Research Achievements in 2016 by Traditional Korean Medicine Journals — National Development Institute of Korean Medicine. [www.nikom.or.kr]

to the Pharmaceutical Affairs Act at the 96th regular session of the National Assembly for the following reason.

"Currently, the medical supply system in South Korea can be classified into traditional Korean medicine, also referred to as the oriental medicine system, and the western medical system. The healthcare agents are classified into doctors, pharmacists, traditional Korean medicine doctors, and herbal pharmacists, where pharmacists and herbal pharmacists are in charge of preparing and dispensing pharmaceutical products or dispensing in combination with herbal medicine. Recently pharmacists often prepare and dispense herbal medicine leading to chaos in the pharmaceutical product distribution system; therefore, the Article 21 (1) of the current law should be supplemented to stipulate the limits of the pharmacists' rights to dispense medicines. This will also prohibit the dispensing of herbal medicines for establishing work order especially, for protecting and fostering traditional Korean medicine, which has been actively researched and developed recently."

Although the above draft of amendment was replaced by the following proposal from the Health and Social Affairs Committee of the National Assembly, the Ministry of Health and Social Affairs had to take follow−up measures.

"The government shall further strengthen supervision to faithfully implement the ban on the random dispensing of herbal medicines by pharmacists., Decided as a supplementary resolution upon passing the amendment to the Pharmaceutical Affairs Act at the 94th regular session of the National Assembly, while preparing comprehensive measures for balanced development of the oriental and western medicines and refraining from adding the herbal medicine preparation to the Korean Pharmacopoeia."

In the end, the Ministry of Health and Social Affairs added the provision to "keep medicine cabinets other than traditional herbal medicine cabinets in pharmacies and keep them clean" as Article 7 (Precautions for management of a pharmacy), Paragraph (1) ⑦ in the amendment to the Enforcement Rules of the Pharmaceutical Affairs Act in March 1980. Resulting in the famous "traditional herbal medicine cabinet" provision. At the time, when dispensing separation was not implemented, the basic principles for dispensing medicines were not observed properly.

In other words, doctors, dentists, and traditional Korean medicine doctors directly dispensed medicines including herbal medicines in addition to medical treatment such as diagnosis and prescription of patients, and pharmacists arbitrarily dispensed all medicines without a prescription from a doctor. This dispensing practice was inevitable at a time when there was an absolute shortage of healthcare workforce, with the undeniable positive effect of quantitative expansion of healthcare supply. However, with a significant increase in the healthcare and pharmaceutical professionals' increased competition in the healthcare and pharmaceutical market, there were frequent conflicting interests between occupations, leading to dispute among occupations over the right to dispense herbal medicine−sparked by the deletion of the "traditional herbal medicine cabinet" provision.

B. Social conflicts caused by conflict between traditional Korean medicine doctors and pharmacists

In March 1993, the Ministry of Health and Social Affairs amended the Enforcement Rules of the Pharmaceutical Affairs Act and deleted the "traditional herbal medicine cabinet" provision, which had been established in March 1980. Traditional Korean medicine doctors strongly opposed the deletion of the "traditional herbal medicine cabinet" provision as a measure to allow pharmacists to handle herbal medicines. Traditional Korean medicine doctors from all over the country gathered in Seoul and held a rally, and eventually, 11 traditional Korean medicine college students across the country refused to attend classes, causing a serious social problem. As a suspicion of lobbying activities by specific interest groups in the process of amending the Enforcement Decree of the Pharmaceutical Affairs Act surfaced, the appraisal authorities began an investigation into the circumstances of the amendment to the Enforcement Rules of the Pharmaceutical Affairs Act from June. Finally, in June, pharmacies across the country protested by collective closures, arguing that the pharmacies could no longer stay blind to the series of incidents.

The Ministry of Health and Social Affairs believed that the root problem of the conflict between traditional Korean medicine doctors and pharmacists was due to the unified system in the pharmaceutical sector. The healthcare sector was divided into traditional Korean medicine and the western medicine. The Ministry of Health and Social Affairs identified the damage in the traditional Korean medicine sector that had been relatively underdeveloped and neglected in health and medical policies. The sense of crisis that the domain was being invaded was worsening the conflicts, and a fundamental solution was through the amendment to the "Pharmaceutical Affairs Act."

Accordingly, in June of the same year, the Ministry of Health and Social Affairs organized the "Committee on Promoting Amendment to the Pharmaceutical Affairs Act" with doctors, dentists, traditional Korean medicine doctors, pharmacists, representatives of consumer and civic groups, and healthcare experts, and attempted to devise a plan to revise the Pharmaceutical Affairs Act. Nevertheless, it was difficult to reach an agreement due to the conflicting interests between the pharmacists and the traditional Korean medicine doctors. At that point, the "Citizens' Coalition for Economic Justice," which participated as a representative of the consumer and civic groups, announced the "Alternative by the Citizens' Coalition for Economic Justice,". The "Mediation Committee to resolve the Conflict between Traditional Korean Medicine Doctors and Pharmacists" was established to foster an agreement between both parties through four meetings with the representatives of the Korean Pharmaceutical Association and the Association of Korean Medicine. This was recorded as an important event in which the civic groups mediated conflicts between the groups with conflicting interests related to healthcare, which was a social concern.

However, this agreement could not be ratified by frontline pharmacists and traditional Korean medicine doctors, and the Korean Pharmaceutical Association took strong measures such as forcing the chairman to resign and return his pharmacist license. As the collective closure of pharmacies continued in some areas, the acting chairman was arrested for violating the Consumer Protection Act and the Fair−Trading Act.

On the other hand, the Ministry of Health and Social Affairs accepted the mediated draft suggestions by the Citizens' Coalition for Economic Justice to announce the final draft of the proposal for the amendment to the Pharmaceutical Affairs Act in October of the same year. And handed in the proposal for the amendment to the "Pharmaceutical Affairs Act" to the National Assembly while the pharmacists kept protesting by group hunger strikes, etc. The amendment proposal was promulgated as Law No. 4731 in January 1994, after some revisions were made by the Health and Social Affairs Committee.

· Preparing the implementation plan for dispensing separation.
· Establishment of a herbal pharmacist system.
· Expanding the managers of herbal medicine wholesalers to pharmacists, herbal pharmacists, herbal pharmaceutical companies, and those who graduated from colleges and universities with a major related to herbal medicine.
· As a transitional measure following the establishment of the herbal pharmacist system, existing pharmacists and students enrolled in pharmacy schools can only dispense herbal medicines according to the prescriptions of traditional Korean medicine doctors or according to the method of prescribing and dispensing herbal medicines set by the Minister of Health and Social Affairs, only if they have passed the herbal medicine dispensing test.

In accordance with the amendment to the "Pharmaceutical Affairs Act," the "Enforcement Decree of Pharmaceutical Affairs Act" and the "Enforcement Rules Pharmaceutical Affairs Act" were revised. In March 1995, the "Regulations on Types and Methods of Herbal Medicine Prescriptions" (the Ministry of Health and Welfare notice), a guidebook for 100 types of herbal medicine prescriptions and preparations, was promulgated, setting the scope of dispensing by herbal pharmacists and pharmacists qualified to dispense herbal medicines without a prescription from traditional Korean medicine doctors.

In addition, in September of the same year, the policy related to the establishment of the College of Herbal Pharmacology was announced. It was stated that the College of Herbal Pharmacology with a total of 40 students would be established in 1996 within the College of Pharmacy at Kyunghee University and Wonkwang University, which were universities with both the College of Korean Medicine and College of Pharmacy. The "Council for Development of Traditional Korean and Herbal Medicine" was established and operated to discuss the development of traditional Korean medicine as well as dispensing separation, and the policy to conduct the herbal medicine dispensing test in December of the same year was announced. However, as there was another conflict of interests between pharmacists and traditional Korean medicine doctors about establishing the Department of Herbal Pharmacology within the College of Pharmacy and conducting oriental medicine, the confrontation between the two parties continued.

In December, 1995, the herbal medicine dispensing test was conducted. Due to the resistance of the pharmacists, only 49 pharmacists took the test, and pharmacy professors among the members of the examination committee did not participate. On the other hand, with the encouragement of the Korean Pharmaceutical Association, about 25,000 pharmacists took the second herbal medicine dispensing pharmacist test held in May, 1996 where the Korean medicine professors protested by leaving the process of making questions for the test. The Association of Korean Medicine then filed a lawsuit claiming that the herbal medicine dispensing test was invalid. Furthermore, the National Institutes of Health, the institution responsible for conducting the test, was blamed for its inadequate management of the test.

The Ministry of Health and Social Affairs announced the "Comprehensive Measures for Herbal Medicine" in May, 1996, under the judgment that the dispute over herbal medicine should come to an end before the second herbal medicine dispensing test. Nevertheless, when expulsion and retention were repeated as the Korean medicine student refused to attend classes in protest, the "Plan for Fostering and Developing Traditional Korean Medicine" was announced again in August. The Ministry of Health and Social Affairs revised the Enforcement Decree of the Pharmaceutical Affairs Act in March, 1997, and introduced a system to only qualify the graduates from the College of Herbal Pharmacology for taking the herbal pharmacist test, thereby bringing an end to the conflict between traditional Korean medicine doctors and pharmacists which had lasted for five years.

3. Policy efforts for the development of traditional Korean medicine

A. Introduction of traditional Korean medicine hospital system and accreditation system

The Ministry of Health and Welfare introduced the traditional Korean medicine hospital system in order to promote the improvement in the quality of healthcare by enhancing the professionalism of medical institutions and to further induce the improvement in the healthcare system such as the rationalization of small to medium−sized hospitals. Traditional Korean medicine clinics were responsible for treating basic diseases, and traditional Korean medicine hospitals provided specialized medical services for specific diseases. Large oriental hospitals were introduced to establish a healthcare delivery system for traditional Korean medicine that satisfied the diverse healthcare needs of the people by setting functions centered on high−level disease treatment as well as education/research activities. Based on the results of designating and operating seven traditional Korean medicine hospitals as pilot institutions since 2007, seven hospitals have been designated as traditional Korean medicine hospitals in 2011 and are in operation.

Meanwhile, the Ministry of Health and Welfare confirmed the accreditation standards for traditional Korean medicine hospitals in August, 2013. The evaluation standards consisted a total of 241 survey items, of which 204 were common survey items. The accreditation system for traditional Korean medicine hospitals applied to all traditional Korean medicine hospitals on a basis of voluntary participation. If a traditional Korean medicine hospital that wanted to receive accreditation applied for accreditation, the Korea Institute for Healthcare Accreditation (KOIHA) assigned a professional investigator to conduct an investigation and report the results to the healthcare institution that applied for accreditation. The accreditation system for traditional Korean medicine hospitals was implemented in January, 2014[92].

---

92) 2013 Traditional Korean Medicine Yearbook − KOIN − People of Traditional Korean Medicine. [www.koin.re.kr]

B. Safety management of herbal medicine

Standard herbal medicine products are supplied through production, cultivation, drying, and processing stages. In the production stage, they are treated as agricultural products and are recognized as herbal medicines (medicines) only after being processed. Owing to these characteristics of herbal medicines, there are frequent cases of forgery or alteration of origin or distribution of herbal medicines not meeting safety and risk standards during the distribution of herbal medicines. To improve the quality of herbal medicine and ensure the reliability and objectivity of herbal medicine, the government implemented the herbal medicine standardization system, installed and operationalized five herbal medicine distribution support facilities.

The simple processing, packaging, and sales system for herbal medicine (self−standardization system), which refers to the act of selling herbal medicine by simple processing and packaging by herbal medicine sales establishments, has been in place since 1996. This allowed farmers to simply process, pack, and sell herbal medicines produced by them without separate quality inspection in accordance with the provision of Article 34, Paragraph (2) of the "Regulations on Supply and Distribution of Herbal Medicines."

The Ministry of Health and Welfare partially relaxed and applied this system in accordance with the long−standing distribution of herbal medicines and the situation of farms growing herbal medicines. In January 2011, the simple processing, packaging, and sales system for herbal medicine was abolished by deleting the provision of the Regulations on Supply and Distribution of Herbal Medicines. This was the basis for the relaxation of the system in order to establish an environment in which only standard herbal medicine products are distributed and used. The system has been fully implemented since April, 2012 after allowing the periods for public relations and emptying the stocks by accepting the suggestions of the herbal medicine industry.

The Ministry of Health and Welfare decided that it was urgent to establish a foundation for fostering and developing the high value−added herbal medicine industry's growth potential and international competitiveness. The herbal medicine distribution support facility was a distribution infrastructure with the functions to maintain constant temperature and constant humidity, installed in five regions (Pyeongchang−gun, Gangwon; Jecheon−si, Chungbuk; Jinan−gun, Jeonbuk; Hwasun−gun, Jeonnam; and Andong−si, Gyeongbuk). These are the main areas of herbal medicine production in South Korea. These facilities were equipped with the equipment for quality inspection, processing, and storage. The construction of the facilities started in July, 2009, and was completed in June, 2010. They are being operated under a subsidy (rent support) project by each local government.

C. Public Health Programs and promoting globalization of traditional Korean medicine

The Ministry of Health and Welfare has been implementing community−based Korean medical public health services since 2001 with public health traditional Korean medicine doctors who were assigned to community health centers in rural areas since 1998. In 2001, for the development of health management programs such as stroke prevention, smoking cessation and acupuncture, four integrated community health centers and five rural fishing villages' community health centers were selected to conduct a pilot project for community−based Korean medical public health services.

In 2002, community—based Korean medical public health services were implemented in connection with the existing health promotion projects. In addition, the traditional Korean medicine health promotion project at the hub community health centers was carried out to provide specialized high—quality traditional Korean medicine health promotion programs such as stroke prevention classes, qigong exercise, and Sasang constitution—based health class. Starting with designated 23 hub community health centers in 2005, the number has been expanded by 15 every year. In 2012, 85 health centers were designated as hub community health centers through government grant of KRW 4,140 million. The department of traditional Korean medicine was established at Suncheon Medical Center in 2006, Cheongju Medical Center in 2007, and Busan Medical Center in 2009 (three departments), with each funded through government grant of KRW 1,311 million, to establish infrastructure for cooperation between western and traditional Korean medicine in the treatment of major chronic and degenerative disease of the elderly such as stroke, diabetes, and hypertension, and to develop a standard cooperation model[93].

In 2013, in line with the integrated promotion of health promotion projects of community health centers, the traditional Korean medicine public health project solve the health problems of local residents, including treatment of chronic degenerative diseases that increased with the aging and to contribute to the improvement of people's health and quality of life by providing traditional Korean medicine health promotion programs suitable for each life cycle.

Considering that 2013 marked the 400th anniversary of the publication of "Donguibogam (Principles and Practice of Eastern Medicine)," the Ministry of Health and Welfare had been carrying out the "project in celebration of the 400th anniversary of the publication of Donguibogam" since 2006 to reinvent traditional Korean medicine and herbal medicine as an international brand. As a result, Donguibogam was registered as a UNESCO Memory of the World for the first time as a medical book. In addition, in order to improve the accessibility and status of traditional Korean medicine in literature, five chapters and 23 books (acupuncture, collecting and prescribing natural medicines, inner body, external appearance, and various diseases) out of a total of 5 chapters 25 books of Donguibogam were translated and published in English. In order to illuminate the life, achievements, and academic values of Jun Heo, six of nine types of medical books (Naeuiseongan, Nabyakjeungchibang, Yukdaeeuihaksungsee, Eonhaeduchangjipyo, Eonhaegugeupbang, and Eonhaetaesanjipyo) were photo—printed and published in Korean.

In recent years, there have been joint efforts and active information exchange to raise international interest in traditional medicine and to develop it into a unique traditional medicine of each country. In this regard, the first attempt was the South Korea—China cooperation project in the field of traditional medicine. At the South Korea—China summit in March 1994, the two countries agreed to promote cooperative projects in the field of traditional medicine, and the exchanges between some private traditional Korean hospitals and research institutes have been made for research and academic exchanges cooperation in standardization fields such as the quality of traditional Korean medicine and Chinese medicine, joint effort on research on incurable diseases and herbal medicines, and inter—company exchange and cooperation were agreed on.

---

93) 10 Major Research Achievements in 2016 by Traditional Korean Medicine Journals — National Development Institute of Korean Medicine. [www.nikom.or.kr]

Currently, WHO is conducting a standardization project related to traditional medicine information and for clinical guidelines. South Korea, has been actively cooperating with the WHO and major participants such as China and Japan to establish international standards in the field of traditional medicine through International Conference on Translational Medicine (ICTM) on disease classification system for traditional Korean medicine. This is based on the WHO International Standard Terminologies on Traditional Medicine (IST−TM)[94].

---

94) Untitled − Korea Institute of Oriental Medicine Webzine. [kiom.e−eyagi.com]

Section 6

Response to New Infectious Diseases and Public Health Crisis

1. Rise of new infectious diseases and policy changes for prevention and control

A. Severe acute respiratory syndrome (SARS)

In September 2003, the World Health Organization (WHO) announced that by the end of the epidemic on July 5, 2003, 8,098 people in 29 countries had been infected and 774 people died, and 21% (1,707) of the patients were healthcare workers. To block the inflow of SARS into South Korea, the government operated a pan−government all−out response system from the early stage of the epidemic (March 16, to July 30, 2003). The Government Joint SARS Countermeasure Headquarters (Prime Minister's Office) and Central SARS Prevention Countermeasure Headquarters (Ministry of Health and Welfare) were established, and all healthcare institutions in South Korea, including the National Institute of Health, National Quarantine Station, and community health centers in cities and provinces (242 centers) maintained a 24−hour emergency system. The government established and operated the SARS Alert system through hospitals and clinics all across the country. The SARS Alert monitoring system was implemented for 998 healthcare institutions by forming a network of 127 emergency healthcare institutions and 47 infection experts nationwide. In addition, SARS was designated as a disease subject for quarantine by amending the Enforcement Rules of the Quarantine Act (May 2, 2003).

As a quarantine measure, follow−up investigations of 230,000 people entering the SARS risk area (temperature measurement and quarantine survey for those entering the risk area through airports and ports: 5,365 aircraft, 614,661 people, 9,513 ships, 276,114 people quarantined) and SARS−related consultations were conducted via phone number 1339. In addition, various guidelines related to SARS prevention and control (for administrative institutions, for healthcare institutions) were produced and distributed, and equipment for prevention and control (75,000 N95 masks, 30,000 protective suits, and 15,000 protective glasses) were distributed to quarantine officers. Through strict quarantine at the initial stage, such as reinforcing public awareness through multiple media, it was possible to prevent the spread of the disease without domestic patients. The government supported medical expenses for suspected patients, designated and operated a total of 41 isolation treatment hospitals (a total of 138 beds) for each region across the country.

B. Avian influenza (AI) human infection

Avian influenza (AI) is a livestock infectious disease that occurs in birds such as wild birds as well as poultry like chickens and ducks due to avian influenza virus (AIV) infection. AI is classified into high and low pathogenicity. Highly pathogenic AI has high risk and is also designated as a disease to be managed by the World Organization for Animal Health (OIE)[95]. Avian influenza virus has a total of 198 different subtypes depending on the combination of proteins located on the surface of the virus, and there are significant differences in the subtypes that can be infected depending on the host type. Accordingly, avian influenza virus generally does not infect humans, but since the 1990s, human infection cases of H5 and H7 types of AI such as A (H5N1) and A (H7N9) have occurred continuously in regions such as Southeast Asia, China, and Egypt. Therefore causing some growing concerns about the emergence of new viruses due to mutations.

Since the first outbreak of the highly pathogenic avian influenza A (H5N1) in poultry in December, 2003 in South Korea, there have been five outbreaks of avian influenza in wild birds and poultry, including avian influenza A (H5N8) that was prevalent in 2006, 2008, 2010, and 2014 to present. Health authorities have produced and distributed publicity materials such as infection prevention leaflets, Q&A booklets, and posters for various groups of people, such as livestock farmers, participants in culling, and local community residents in the avian influenza outbreak areas while striving to deliver the right information about avian influenza in a timely manner through distribution of press releases and interviews with media companies.

In order to recognize and diagnose the occurrence of domestic avian influenza patients at an early stage, the National Institute of Health and the Public Health and Research Institute for Control of Infectious Disease established an avian influenza diagnostic testing system and strengthened the monitoring system for healthcare institutions. In addition, the quarantine measures have been reinforced in preparation for the influx of patients from infected countries such as China. And also promotional activities have been carried out to guide overseas travelers on infection prevention rules, and providing behavioral guidelines. Since securing the H5N1 type AI virus strain for vaccine manufacturing in 2007 to develop a pre-pandemic vaccine derived from fertilized eggs in preparation for the H1N1 influenza pandemic. A non-clinical material production process was established, and a domestic product license has been obtained through the non-clinical/clinical phase-1, 2, and 3 trials.

C. Novel swine-origin influenza A (H1N1) in 2009

On April 28, 2009, when the first suspected case occurred in South Korea, the national crisis level was raised from the "concern level" to the "caution level", and the national emergency response system was activated. By mid-August, the epidemic

---

95) Current Status of New Infectious Disease Infection Control and Countermeasures — Medical Device Newsline. [www.kmdianews.com]

standard (2.67 cases per 1,000 people) was exceeded through rapid community spread in early October. After, the national crisis level was raised from the alert level to the severe level in November, 2009, and the number of deaths in South Korea was estimated at 270 before it was lowered back to the concern level in March, 2010. Based on the H1N1 influenza pandemic crisis level set by the WHO, sporadic and small−scale outbreaks of patients were classified as a concern level, outbreaks in a community as a caution level, outbreaks in two or more countries within the same WHO region as a warning level, and outbreaks in several WHO regions as a serious level.

First, in the concern−to−caution level (April 27, 2009 to July 20, 2009), following the occurrence of the first suspected case in South Korea on April 27, 2009, the Korea Centers for Disease Control and Prevention (KCDC) started operating the "Central Disease Control Headquarters." On April 30, the "Central SI Countermeasure Headquarters" was established with the Minister of Health, Welfare and Family Affairs as the Director and the Centers for Disease Control and Prevention, and the National Quarantine Station operated a 24−hour emergency service system. To block the entry of infected patients into the country at the beginning of the epidemic, quarantine measures were strengthened by subjecting all passengers to fever monitoring at entry at the airport (a total of 11.57 million people were quarantined by the end of the epidemic). In addition, for early detection of the patients in the local community, a telephone follow−up survey was conducted for all people entering the risk area (760,000 people including foreigners), and a follow−up survey was conducted for passengers on the same flight upon identifying confirmed cases (3,277 people). In addition, presumed/confirmed cases were quarantined and treated with antiviral drugs through state−designated inpatient treatment centres (197 beds in five hospitals). In addition to promoting infection prevention education for immigrants, a daily reporting system for elementary, middle, and high schools and primary medical institutions (approximately 10,000) was operated to actively monitor acute febrile respiratory illness in the local community.

Then, the situation worsened to the caution level (July 21, 2009 to November 2, 2009) as the epidemic spread in several countries in the Pacific region, it was raised to the alert level. In the beginning, in order to respond to a large−scale outbreak of patients, the existing quarantine and isolation−centered response strategies were switched to damage minimization strategies focusing on patient monitoring and early treatment to lower the rate and scale of the epidemic and to minimize the occurrence of severe cases and deaths.

As a result, treatment base hospitals for each city and province (533 nationwide, about 10,000 beds) were designated, national stockpile of antiviral drugs and personal protective equipment were supplied, healthcare institutions for influenza clinical specimen monitoring were expanded from 678 to 826 institutions, and the confirmation testing system was extended to private healthcare institutions to increase the role of private healthcare institutions. In August, the middle of the alert phase, 240,000 antiviral drugs were distributed to public health centers, treatment hospitals, and base pharmacies. From September, antiviral drug administration and prescription were made available at all healthcare institutions and base pharmacies. In October, the dosing standards were relaxed at all healthcare institutions and all pharmacies to allow antiviral drugs to be prescribed and administered under the judgment of the doctor to all patients with acute febrile respiratory illness with an intention to minimize the occurrence of serious patients through active medication (about 3.58 million patients were administered by June, 2010). Vaccination subjects were selected (39% of the total population, 19.13 million people) considering the infection blocking effect, the risk of infection as major factors, and sequential vaccinations were performed from October 27, 2009, starting with healthcare workers. To improve the effectiveness of the vaccination program, the vaccination reservation system as well as education at consigned healthcare institutions and adverse reaction management system was operated. Upon entering the severe level (November 3, 2009 to December 10, 2009) following the epidemic spread around the world, in November, 2009, with a focus on establishing an emergency response system for critically ill patients and early completion of schools' vaccinations, started on November 11, and healthcare responses aiming at treating patients with severe symptoms such as pneumonia and reducing the number of deaths. By July 31, 2010, 12.89 million people (14.76 million cases) had been vaccinated. Lastly, it was followed by the downgrade of the crisis level and recovery (December 11, 2009 to April 1, 2010). After the severe level, the national crisis level was downgraded to the alert level on December 11, 2009, the caution level on March 8, 2010, and the concern level on April 1, 2010 with a decrease in the number of H1N1 influenza patients. Although the national crisis level was downgraded, free administration of antiviral drugs from the national stockpile was conducted until the end of April in order to minimize the confusion of the public while allowing the preparation period for the distribution of antiviral drugs in the market. Clinical and laboratory monitoring of influenza virus and publicity of hygiene rules such as hand washing were conducted continuously throughout the year[96].

D. Progress of the MERS crisis in 2015

Middle East Respiratory Syndrome (MERS) is an acute respiratory infection caused by a coronavirus. Since MERS cases were first reported in Saudi Arabia in September 2012, a total of 1,499 cases occurred until March 2016. The World Health Organization (WHO) held an emergency meeting on MERS from July 2013 to February 2015, recommending its member states to prepare in advance MERS research and preventive measures against infectious diseases. The United States Centers for Disease Control and Prevention (CDC) identified a high rate of infection among healthcare workers through a joint research with Saudi Arabia and emphasized infection control in hospitals.

In Korea, the Public Health Crisis Response Division was established at the Korea Center for Disease Control and Prevention after the 2009 H1N1 Influenza A (H1N1) pandemic. Nam−soon Kim (2016)[97] in 2014, after the outbreak of MERS, set up a disease control countermeasures team at the infectious disease crisis 'alert level' of concern and the "MERS Prevention and Management Guidelines" created, and revised in December. In June, 2014, the Public Health Crisis Response Project Group held a forum under the theme of "Preparing and Response to the Influx of Middle East Respiratory Syndrome (MERS) in South Korea," that involved experts and officials from

---

96) Ministry of Health and Welfare, "70 Years of Health and Welfare" Volume 2 Healthcare Edition, 2016.

97) Nam−soon Kim (2016), 2015 MERS White Paper What We Learned from MERS!

the Korea Centers for Disease Control and Prevention. In this forum, the prevalence of in－hospital MERS infections was discussed, but no specific preparations were made. Fortunately, after the 2009 H1N1 influenza pandemic, a certain number of negative pressure isolation beds necessary for treating patients with infectious diseases as well as diagnostic technologies for MERS were prepared[98].

Even though there was insufficient preparation for in－hospital MERS infection control in South Korea, economic and cultural exchanges with the Middle East continued to increase. A 68－year－old man running a horticultural business who had visited the Middle East on April 24, 2015 for two weeks before returning home was diagnosed as the first confirmed case of MERS. Through epidemiological study of MERS patients, the index patient spoke with a local purchaser during a visit to the Middle East, but never had contact with camels or ingested food related to camels. The first patient had body aches and fever seven days after returning home and was treated at the clinic, but the symptoms did not improve. At the recommendation of the attending physician, the patient was hospitalized at Pyeongtaek St. Mary's Hospital for three days. The patient showing symptoms of high fever and shortness of breath, visited another clinic, and was admitted to a single room at Samsung Medical Center on May 18. Finally, the doctor in charge considered the patient's travel history to the Middle East, and on May 19, requested the MERS test from the Korea Centers for Disease Control and Prevention. The National Institute of Health conducted a diagnostic test on the respiratory specimen, and the MERS coronavirus gene was detected and reported on May 20[99].

The patient visited several hospitals and clinics for 10 days after the onset of symptoms, and had contact with family members, other patients, and healthcare workers, resulting in a number of secondary transmission. The indexed patient was transferred to the National Medical Center and treated in an isolation ward. As the wife of the first patient was diagnosed to be infected, treated at the same hospital.

After the first confirmed case of MERS on May 20, 2015, the Korea Centers for Disease Control and Prevention raised the infectious disease crisis alert from "concern" to "caution" as specified in the "Standard Manual for Infectious Disease Crisis Management". The Central Disease Control Headquarters was established at the Korea Centers for Disease Control and Prevention, and quarantine measures was strengthened for those entering the Middle East. The National Institute of Health formed a health team that operated a 24－hour dedicated MERS testing and informed the World Health Organization (WHO) of the MERS outbreak. The Central Disease Control Headquarters announced that all close contacts with the first patient who had the possibility of infection, had been identified.

In the initial epidemiological investigation, the criteria for judging a close contact with a high probability of infection were 1) a person who had physical contact with a confirmed or suspected patient, or 2) a person who stayed together in a space within 2m for more than one hour while the patient was symptomatic. The Central Disease Control Headquarters applied these standards to the indexed patient and

---

98) MERS White Paper － Gyeonggi－do Infectious Disease Control Headquarters. [www.gidcc.or.kr]
99) Seong－do Lee (2017) A Study of Crisis Communication in Korea: The Case S study on MERS Epidemic, Chungbuk National University, August 2017. 8.

conducted isolation of close contacts. At Pyeongtaek St. Mary's Hospital, measures were taken to isolate only patients who were admitted to the same room with the first patient, healthcare workers, and moved other patients to the ward on the seventh floor (Joon−seo Lee, 2018)[100] Different from the expectations of the Central Disease Control Headquarters, the sixth patient had not been admitted to the same ward as the indexed patient but was confirmed to be infected on May 28, 2015. These were followed by additional confirmed cases. In addition, the daughter of the third patient did not have fever by May 20 and was not subjected to quarantine. She was diagnosed as a confirmed case a few days later. In addition, there was an incident where a close contact was not quarantined, left the country and was confirmed with MERS by the Chinese health authorities.

In the process of investigating the MERS epidemic at Pyeongtaek St. Mary's Hospital, the infectivity of the MERS virus was found to be different. Therefore, to reduce the possibility of MERS virus transmission as much as possible, the exposure period of "one hour" was deleted from the criteria for determining close contacts. As there were confirmed cases that did not meet the fever criteria of 38.0°C, the criterion was changed to 37.5°C or higher for the purpose of early detection.

As the MERS epidemic spread, it was necessary to completely revise the previously established quarantine strategy. The Ministry of Health and Welfare convened the Infectious Disease Crisis Management Countermeasure Committee on May 28 2015, and completely reorganized the MERS response system. The first key to reorganizing the MERS response system was by forming the "Central MERS Management Countermeasures Headquarters" as a new response organization with the Ministry of Health and Welfare overseeing the overall response. The Centers for Disease Control and Prevention oversaw quarantine, epidemiological investigation and diagnosis. Secondly, a policy was established to review the epidemiological investigation process using private experts related to infectious diseases and disease epidemiology and to flexibly apply the response manual and various guidelines. Thirdly, government−wide support was provided to prepare to respond to MERS.

The Central MERS Management Countermeasures Headquarters continued to expand and reorganize the response system. To respond to in−hospital infections, a public−private comprehensive response TF was formed on June 4, 2015, and an immediate response team was organized on June 8 according to the President's instructions. The immediate response team was in charge of immediately recommending the necessary measures to prevent the spread of infection in a specific hospital as a top priority. The epidemiological investigation team of the Central MERS Management Countermeasures Headquarters had a central private epidemiological investigation support group under the Korean Society for Preventive Medicine, and private epidemiological investigation support teams were organized in cities and provinces.

To provide pan−governmental support to the Central MERS Management Countermeasures Headquarters, 11 ministries and local governments, started operating from June 3, 2015. Minister of Public Safety and Security acted as the director of the Pan−governmental MERS Countermeasure Support Headquarters, with the participation of the Office for Government Policy Coordination, Ministry of Health and Welfare,

---

100) Joon−seo Lee (2018), A Study on Improvement of Infectious Disease Control and Prevention Act and System.

Education, Foreign Affairs, National Defense, Government Administration and Home Affairs, Culture, Sports and Tourism, Agriculture, Food and Rural Affairs, Oceans and Fisheries, and the National Police Agency.

While the central government was reorganizing the quarantine strategy and response system, the MERS outbreak occurred at Samsung Medical Center. A 35−year−old male who was hospitalized with pneumonia symptoms at Pyeongtaek St. Mary's Hospital visited the emergency room of Samsung Medical Center and was confirmed as the 14th MERS patient. The 14th MERS patient had contact with many people in a crowded emergency room environment, and dozens of secondary infections occurred. Samsung Medical Center sent a list of exposed persons to the Ministry of Health and Welfare in the early morning of May 31, but the entire list of exposed persons was not provided at once. In the process of identifying close contacts, the range of movement within the hospital was not sufficiently considered, and a confirmed case appeared among those who were excluded from the contact list. As people who were not in the same room as the first confirmed case at Pyeongtaek St. Mary's Hospital were diagnosed as a confirmed case, false alarm began to spread rapidly on the Internet and social network services (SNS) from the end of May.

The government revealed that the alarm lacked grounds through Twitter and other SNS and provided factual information related to the stories by using portal Q&As, knowledge encyclopedias, content search corners, and started regular briefings on June 1, 2015. However, the public's distrust increased due to the inability to respond in timely to matters that the public was curious about, such as the disclosure of the name of the medical institutions where the confirmed cases occurred and where the confirmed cases visited.

The public anxiety about the MERS outbreak and the demand for information disclosure about healthcare institutions where confirmed MERS patients emerged grew. The Central MERS Management Countermeasures Headquarters decided to provide information on areas related to confirmed cases, names of medical institutions, and exposure dates through a public−private joint task force meeting, that was limited to "infectious diseases specialists and the infection control office." On June 3, 2015, there was an instruction to promptly and transparently disclose MERS−related information at a public−private joint emergency inspection meeting presided by the president.

Meanwhile, there was conflicts over the management of quarantined persons between the central and local governments. At a night briefing on June 4, 2015, without prior consultation with the Ministry of Health and Welfare, the Seoul Metropolitan Government disclosed that the 35th patient, a doctor from Samsung Medical Center, attended the housing association general assembly, and demanded for voluntary self−isolation for those who attended the housing association general assembly. On the other hand, the Central MERS Management Countermeasures Headquarters expressed the opinion that the 35th patient's transmission risk was low, so the degree of contact of the participants of the housing association general assembly should be classified for management.

The Central MERS Management Countermeasures Headquarters discussed the need for preemptive quarantine measures at the MERS−Public−Private Comprehensive TF Meeting and disclosed the hospital name of Pyeongtaek St. Mary's Hospital on June 5. Afterwards, through a joint meeting with the heads of local governments, it was agreed to promote the disclosure of the second medical institution, and on June 7, 2015, the names of 24 medical institutions were disclosed. After the disclosure of information on medical institutions, measures such as the establishment of screening clinics and operation of the National Safety Hospitals were announced one after another. The MERS hotline was operated, and prevention rules and precautions for hospital use were publicized in schools and public places.

The infectious disease crisis alert due to the MERS outbreak was at the level of "caution," but the response went beyond that. As the organization of the Central MERS Management Countermeasure Headquarters was reorganized and the direction of the public−private comprehensive response TF became clear, the national level public−private cooperation response system was put into action in earnest. To relieve public anxiety about MERS and to adjust all policies related to quarantine, the acting prime minister hosted the Pan−governmental Countermeasures Meetings from June 9, 2015. Major local governments, in line with the central government, rectified the shortcomings of the first reaction organization and built a response system adequate for contact isolation and management.

Many employees of the Ministry of Health and Welfare and related ministries were assigned to the Central MERS Management Countermeasures Headquarters. Approximately 250 persons participated in the MERS response, including those conducting similar activities without joining the headquarters. The immediate response team of the public−private comprehensive response TF was dispatched to the medical institution where the MERS patient occurred, inspected the site and supervised the immediate response.

In the early stages of the MERS outbreak, patients were to be isolated and treated in the existing state−designated inpatient treatment (isolation) facilities and negative pressure isolation beds secured at base hospitals by cities and provinces. With the increase in the number of patients, there was a shortage of negative pressure isolation beds in Seoul, Gyeonggi, Daejeon, and Chungcheong regions. To overcome this, MERS central medical institutions and infectious disease management institutions were designated to expand negative pressure isolation beds in the short term, Portable negative pressure devices and negative pressure tents were purchased and supplied to infectious disease management organizations. Demand for equipment needed to treat severe MERS patients increased, but there was no enough supply. The National Medical Center surveyed the demand for personal protective and treatment equipment, while the Central MERS Management Countermeasures Headquarters provided related equipment to intensive management hospitals.

The Central MERS Management Countermeasures Headquarters tried to disclose all matters to the public as transparently as possible to satisfy the public needs for information, and to carry out quarantine measures smoothly. The government's regular MERS briefing continued until July 17, 2015, as organized data on the MERS outbreak and management measures were provided to all media. The MERS portal (www.mers.go.kr) is an information window that collects published data in one place, providing major issues such as operation of medical institutions with confirmed cases, screening clinics and national safety hospitals, and treatment guidelines. The 24−hour MERS hotline (109) played a major role as a civil complaint window where the public could ask questions if they had any suspicious symptoms or questions.

The "Infectious Disease Control and Prevention Act" was partially amended to solve the problems revealed during the MERS response. The amendment to the law allowed the designation of new, overseas infectious diseases that have not yet been introduced into South Korea as class 4 infectious diseases. In addition, the rights and obligations of the central and local governments, healthcare workers and institutions, and citizens for the prevention and control of infectious diseases have been strengthened. The law stipulated the authority of quarantine officers and epidemiological investigators, which was a problem in responding to MERS, and laid the groundwork for collecting information necessary for patient management and cooperating. The reporting obligations of institutions where infectious disease pathogens were found were stipulated, and it was specified to prepare an information system for the prevention and control.

It was also noteworthy that the legal grounds for mandatory quarantine, etc. to control and manage those who were likely to spread the infectious disease, as well as the grounds for punishment of acts that interfere with the quarantine work, such as false statements at medical institutions, were prepared. To compensate for the economic disadvantages of quarantined and hospitalized persons, the National Assembly operated the "Committee on Special Countermeasures for Middle East Respiratory Syndrome (MERS)". Following this, there was established legal grounds for patients who were isolated to be compensated and that incorporated paid leave, treatment cost, living support and other financial support. Health care institutions were also compensated for their loss. The "Committee on Special Countermeasures for Middle East Respiratory Syndrome (MERS)" pointed out that the causes of the outbreak included the lack of initial response by the quarantine authorities, delay in information disclosure, confusion of control agencies, and insufficient establishment of cooperation between the central government, local governments, and private healthcare institutions. In addition, the problems of insufficient infrastructure related to infectious diseases of the Ministry of Health and Welfare and the Korea Centers for Disease Control and Prevention, including facility structure and hospital preparedness, as well as the culture of healthcare use were identified as causes.

The infectious disease control measures presented by the "Committee on Special Countermeasures for Middle East Respiratory Syndrome (MERS)" included: 1) improvement of organizational problems of the Korea Centers for Disease Control and Prevention, 2) improvement of quarantine manual, 3) authorization necessary and flexible response by quarantine officers, 4) expansion of professional manpower, facilities and equipment, and international cooperation, 5) improvement of medical delivery system and usage culture, and 6) national compensation for social costs caused by MERS (patients, healthcare workers, quarantined persons and healthcare institutions). The Board of Audit and Inspection announced the results of its audit on MERS prevention and response in January 2016. The Board of Audit and Inspection pointed out the neglect of research and guideline establishment in preparation for the MERS response and pointed out problems such as the failure to follow-up monitoring after the epidemiological investigation of the first patient in the initial response. For the third confirmed case, which did not fit the characteristics of droplet infection, investigation and analysis should have been carried out on ventilation holes in relation to the cause of infection and the route of infection. The failure to preemptively review the disclosure of medical institution information was pointed out as a problem. Furthermore, it was pointed out that an error occurred in the process of securing the 14th patient's list of close contacts in the steps taken by Samsung Medical Center for MERS patients, and that the submission of the contact list by Samsung Medical Center was delayed.

Based on the results of the audit, the Board of Audit and Inspection requested to improve the issues of securing full-time employees to strengthen the capabilities of the Korea Centers for Disease Control and Prevention, regularization of epidemiological investigators not even properly discussed, and the insufficient "infectious disease management action plan" at metropolitan and regional governments. In addition, the education and training for in−hospital infection, improvement of medical institution facility standards and medical institution certification system were necessary.

The Board of Audit and Inspection pointed out a total of 39 cases [eight disciplinary cases (16 people), 13 cautions, and 18 notices] targeting 18 institutions including the Ministry of Health and Welfare and the Korea Centers for Disease Control and Prevention and demanded disciplinary action against those involved. On the other hand, regarding the request for disciplinary action by the Board of Audit and Inspection, it was impossible to attribute the limitations of the system and environment to personal faults, and there was "hindsight bias" as some items pointed out were uncertain at the time, but only became clear after the epidemic ended.

The MERS Follow−up Action TF conducted interviews with on−site experts to prepare recovery measures and held a public hearing on the reorganization of the national quarantine system. In relation to the reorganization of the national quarantine system, the Infectious Disease Control Committee, government−ruling party consultations, national policy coordination meetings were held to collect and coordinate opinions from various fields, and in September 2015, a plan for the national quarantine system reform was proposed. The 48 tasks in the plan for the national quarantine system reform included: 1) strengthening the capabilities of the Korea Centers for Disease Control and Prevention, 2) governance and cooperation system for emerging infectious diseases, 3) tasks to improve quarantine, and 4) strengthening the infection control capacity of hospitals, improving facilities, and changing hospital−visiting culture.

The MERS epidemic was not controlled with genetic technology or advanced medicines, but ended by traditional quarantine measures such as epidemiological investigation, isolation, and quarantine. Therefore, both the central and local governments recognized the need for a "public health organization and workforce".

To respond to a new infectious disease, a manual based on the latest knowledge was needed, and training based on desk theory was insufficient to deal with the situation. During the response process, it was necessary to quickly analyze the crisis.

As seen in the MERS epidemic, the primary response to infectious diseases took place in the local community, and those under quarantine had to be managed by the local government. Therefore, there was increased awareness that local governments needed an "infectious disease control organization" expertise for autonomous response.

As the crowded environment of hospitals acted as a factor in the spread of infectious diseases, structural problems in the healthcare systems' vulnerability to infectious diseases had to be addressed. After the MERS outbreak, many healthcare workers became aware of new infectious diseases and recognized that healthcare−related infections were of public health concern.

The conflict between the Korea Centers for Disease Control and Prevention (Ministry of Health and Welfare) and local governments caused confusion in urgent situations, and the lack of partnership between public health authorities and healthcare institutions was also a problem. Therefore, the necessity of establishing an "infectious disease response network" among the Korea Centers for Disease Control and Prevention, local governments and healthcare institutions were suggested. After MERS, the public realized the importance of preventive measures such as wearing a mask in preventing infectious diseases as well as the risk of infection in the process of using hospitals and clinics, including emergency rooms. The people became aware of the need to comply with infectious disease prevention rules and cooperate in improving the culture of healthcare use (Nam-soon Kim, 2016)[101].

2. Application of policies for response to new infectious diseases through COVID-19

A. Initial response

Domestic infectious disease experts immediately began a risk assessment when the government heard the news that pneumonia of unknown cause had occurred in China. The government's initial response was evaluated as positive considering the smooth progress from strengthening quarantine to setting up a screening clinic, identifying patients, and quarantine of contacts.

Considering that indexed patient was immediately quarantined at the airport after the outbreak of COVID-19 and that patient 2 was also classified as a subject of active surveillance during the quarantine process and was monitored by the health authorities, it was evaluated that the quarantine response was well performed to prevent the spread in the early stage.

Nevertheless, the Korean Medical Association evaluated the government's initial response as negative since the ban on entry from China was not implemented and resulted in South Korea to becoming the world's second-largest COVID-19 outbreak country after China. The Korean Medical Association criticized the government for not accepting the recommendations of the Association to ban entry from China despite the request made six times.

In addition, there were negative public opinions on the initial response that expectations for premature end to COVID-19 led to the spread of infection, that provision of travel history to third countries other than China was not implemented promptly, and that the excessive anxiety of the people was not properly addressed. However, at the end of the day, it was evaluated to be in tandem with the democratic and open policy of the government.

B. Large-scale diagnostic tests

As of April 1 2020, the cumulative number of COVID-19 tests was about 430,000, with up to 30,000 tests possible per day. The Korea Centers for Disease Control and Prevention (KCDC) conducted 5,000 to 6,000 tests per day. In Daegu, about 68,000 diagnostic tests were conducted, and more than half of them (37,000) were mobile tests in which public health doctors directly visited the homes or hospitals of symptomatic or suspected patients to collect samples.

Many people gave a positive evaluation of the diagnostic capability and crisis management of the Korea Centers for Disease Control and Prevention for these mass tests. South Korea's excellent diagnostic capabilities such as rapid diagnosis of COVID-19 and data acquisition were also highly evaluated internationally. There were also positive reviews for

---

101) Nam-soon Kim (2016), 2015 MERS White Paper What We Learned from MERS!

approving the test kit developed by a private company and taking measures to allow testing anywhere in the country by creating temporary screening stations such as drive−through and walk−through screening stations.

As the Korea Centers for Disease Control and Prevention conducted a large−scale diagnostic test, the number of confirmed COVID−19 cases initially seemed to increase rapidly, but as a result, it helped early detection. By providing prompt treatment and medical help, the fatality rate in South Korea was as low as 0.71%. There was an opinion that large amounts of data were gathered from such preventive measures, helping authorities focus on mass infections in quarantine measures and virus tracking as well as the assessment of infection density.

However, there were also criticisms of excessive testing. There was a negative evaluation that thorough mass testing as well as treatment and quarantine measures conducted even for those with mild symptoms resulted in a surge of confirmed cases leading to a shortage of beds and confusion in healthcare institutions, thereby collapsing the healthcare infrastructure, causing inability to accept seriously ill patients. In general, it was positively evaluated as a preventive diagnostic testing scheme that contributed to early stabilization.

C. Disclosure of information on confirmed cases and privacy

Positions on information disclosure and invasion of privacy are still sharply divergent. It is necessary to disclose the movement for the purpose of public interest for the safety of the community as the sacrifice of individual rights for the protection of the health of many is. Compared to Europe and the United States, which did not provide reliable information due to individual human rights issues, South Korea's transparent and open information disclosure was positively evaluated as it was helpful in terms of respecting the people's right to know, preventing the spread of infectious diseases, and managing the infection.

In addition, there was an opinion that information disclosure was a necessary quarantine measure allowing residents to take a preemptive response in a situation with a rapidly spreading epidemic.

Nevertheless, there was an ongoing criticism that such a disclosure of information was an invasion of privacy. Negative public opinion emerged that transparent information disclosure, a characteristic of democratic quarantine, would infringe individual human rights for the sake of public interest. Although it was necessary to disclose the route of the confirmed cases, an excessive scope of disclosure such as detailed travel routes (times) and places of visit, gender, birth year, nationality, visit to Wuhan, entry date, confirmation date, and information on hospitalization and healthcare institution could lead to a serious invasion of privacy for the confirmed cases.

Although information that could identify the confirmed cases, such as name, phone number, or address, was not posted on the website, there was a possibility of human rights violations as the detailed movement routes and sensitive information of COVID−19 confirmed cases were disclosed on SNS and the website. In addition, there was criticism that only the information necessary to prevent infection should be disclosed as it was possible for acquaintances or co−workers to infer the work location and movement information of the confirmed cases. In fact, whenever the path of movement of the N−th confirmed case was revealed, baseless speculations and slanders such as "Why did you go to the hotel?" and "Wandering around like a rogue" were rampant on the Internet. As the members of the Shincheonji Church were attached to the confirmed cases who visited Daegu regardless of the date or purpose of the visit, unnecessary information disclosure was pointed out to cause an adverse effect, inducing some people with symptoms to hide, out of fear of revealing their movements.

D. Immigration control of infected persons

From March 22, the government conducted a diagnostic test for COVID−19 on all inbound travelers from Europe, and those with symptoms were asked to wait in an airport quarantine facility and undergo a diagnostic test. Those without symptoms were moved to a facility for screening. Those tested negative were subjected to self−quarantine for 14 days and follow−up management through active monitoring before returning home. For those arriving from the United States, diagnostic tests were conducted only when symptoms appeared after quarantine at a facility. However, as the number of confirmed cases of COVID−19 increased, the government mandated that all those arriving from the United States and those arriving from Europe be tested within three days of self−quarantine regardless of symptoms after entering South Korea, from April 13. For foreigners entering South Korea for a short−term stay, the same level of quarantine management measures as in Europe was considered. It was planned to first conduct a diagnostic test at an open screening clinic installed in the airport and then place them under quarantine at a temporary residential facility for 14 days.

To prevent re−entry of the virus into the country, strong measures was carried out for new entries by operating express buses and KTX−only cars to separate their movement lines. Regarding the government's diagnostic testing and monitoring of inbound travelers, there was a positive evaluation that it was an active response. On the other hand, there was also a critical opinion. Currently, with close to 10,000 people visiting South Korea a day, paying the national treasury for COVID−19 diagnostic tests, treatment, and management regardless of the nationality was criticized as a quarantine model that looks like shoveling sand against the tide. In addition, there was a public opinion that there was a risk of insufficient screening capacity due to excessive and unnecessary testing and even a concern that an infected foreigner might board a flight to South Korea for treatment with the continuous inflow from overseas unless their entry was banned.

E. Problems associated with mask distribution and mask wearing

When a shortage of masks and a sell−out problem occurred following the outbreak of COVID−19, the government intervened directly in production and distribution of masks led by the Ministry of Food and Drug Safety. The proportion of masks purchased and distributed by the government was expanded to 80% of the total production. After that, as a countermeasure against the unstable supply and demand in line with the surge, a five−day rotation public face mask distribution system was introduced allowing people to purchase masks on the day corresponding to the last digit of their birth year.

The government−led public mask distribution policy was positively evaluated in South Korea and overseas. It was evaluated as a traditional solution that guaranteed fairness while resolving shortcomings. In addition, the strong public mask policy of the South Korean government and the strong sharing of sales information by pharmacies were analyzed to be the secret to a smooth supply of masks. The mask distribution system of the South Korean government, which strongly controlled the price and supply of masks, was highly praised.

However, some expressed doubts as to whether the public mask policy to prevent the sell−off and the surge in the mask market was being properly observed. There was also criticism that it was efficient to distribute public masks for free or to distribute them at each community center. There was a negative evaluation of the government's lack of problem−solving ability pointing out the high price of the public mask at KRW 1,500, compared to that of Taiwan at KRW 200; the unrealistic proxy purchase method; the socialist distribution system; and the inability to solve the mask problem because South Korea was ranked fifth in the world in manufacturing and second in mask production capacity.

F. Operation of the quarantine response governance system
(1) Central government level

South Korea's COVID−19 quarantine response system consisted of the Central Disease Control (Korea Centers for Disease Control and Prevention), the Central Disaster and Safety Countermeasure, the Central Disaster Management under the Ministry of Health and Welfare, and the Pan−governmental Support under the Ministry of Public Administration and Security, in cooperation with Local Disaster and Safety Countermeasure Headquarters under each local government. On February 23, 2020, after the onset of the COVID−19, the government raised the infectious disease crisis level to severe and activated the Central Disaster and Safety Countermeasure Headquarters, led by the Prime Minister.

The Central Disease Control Headquarters (Korea Centers for Disease Control and Prevention), as a quarantine control tower, took over the roles of preparing and taking measures as well as monitoring and briefing on the current situation. The Central Disaster and Safety Countermeasure Headquarters (Prime Minister) strengthened the government−wide response and support system between the central and local governments. The Central Disaster Management Headquarters (Ministry of Health and Welfare) supported the prevention of the spread of infection in the community and the quarantine work of the Central Disease Control. The Pan−governmental Support Headquarters (Ministry of Public Administration and Security) supported necessary matters such as cooperation between the central and local governments, response support, and operation of temporary residential facilities.

Each local government also formed the "Local Disaster and Safety Countermeasure Headquarters" led by the governor to ensure the provision of infectious disease hospitals and beds for the establishment of a regional quarantine system. They also played a role in supporting resources such as beds, manpower, and materials.

In addition, the National Crisis Management Center (National Security Office) served as a security control tower; the Central Clinical Committee (National Medical Center) provided support for epidemiological investigations as well as research support; the University/International Student COVID−19 support group (Ministry of Education) provided support for the response of city and provincial offices of education, the status and management of international students entering South Korea; and the Special Committee on COVID−19 Countermeasures (National Assembly Health and Welfare Committee) revised and institutionalized laws related to infectious diseases.

(2) Local government level

As the number of confirmed cases of COVID−19 in Daegu, Gyeonbuk, increased, the government formed a pan−governmental special countermeasure support group (hereafter referred to as the pan−governmental support group) and dispatched it to Daegu to prevent the spread of the disease.

The pan−governmental support group was centered on the Central Disaster Management Headquarters, consisting of the operational team with the Ministry of Public Administration and Security and the National Police Agency, the healthcare support team with the Ministry of Welfare and the Fire Department, the departmental cooperation team with Ministry of Environment and three other departments, the local government liaison team with Daegu and Gyeonbuk local governments, and the press response team (Jong−Goo Lee, 2002)[102].

From February 20, the pan−governmental support group played the roles including supporting the Central Disaster Management Headquarters, coordination of work between relevant ministries and local governments, commanding the Director of the Local Disaster and Safety Countermeasure Headquarters, dispatching, and managing pan−governmental support groups for cities and provinces, and self−quarantine and response support at the local government level. In addition, it took on the role of taking necessary measures on site, such as providing medical and quarantine supplies, self−quarantine management and supporting relief supplies, workplace quarantine, employment stability support, and waste disposal.

From February 26, the Prime Minister, who was the Director of the Central Disaster Management Headquarters, visited Daegu, where many people were infected with COVID−19, and took the lead in quarantine activities. While staying in Daegu for 19 days until March 13, the Prime Minister presided over Central Disaster Management Headquarters meetings at Daegu City Hall every morning, established residential treatment centers through phone calls to companies to overcome the shortage of beds, and took charge of on−site management to promptly respond to and resolve requests for support in the region.

(3) Establishment of cooperation system

After the spread of COVID−19, the government took a pan−governmental response by establishing a cooperative system among related ministries and local governments. The National Police Agency and the Ministry of Justice used related information systems to quickly identify contacts, while the Ministry of Land, Infrastructure and Transport and the Ministry of Culture, Sports and Tourism supported communication and cooperation with the private sector, such as airlines and the travel industry. In addition, the Ministry of Foreign Affairs organized an emergency response team centered on the Overseas Safety Guard Center and maintained a 24−hour response system under an organic cooperative system with diplomatic offices and related ministries overseas.

The Ministry of Education established a cooperative system with universities and local governments to share information on inbound international students, conducted intensive quarantine in universities, temporary residences, densely populated areas, and formed a joint response group for international students from China.

---

102) Jong−Goo Lee (2002), A Study on the Establishment of Strategies for Responding to the Resurgence of COVID−19.

The government supported urgent research in cooperation with industry, academia, research circles, and hospitals to develop COVID−19 treatments and vaccines, and supported the open use of core resources such as research facilities, pathogen resources and clinical data.

The people also participated in the cooperation between the government and each local government. Office workers voluntarily returned part of their salaries, and building owners reduced or exempted rent for the business owners and tenants.

G. Healthcare system (the role of National Health Insurance)

In South Korea's healthcare system for infectious diseases, the government, the National Health Insurance Corporation, and local governments jointly bear all the expenses necessary for screening, isolation, and treatment in accordance with the Infectious Disease Control and Prevention Act.

Among medical expenses, reimbursed items, patient co−payments, and food and medical costs for inpatient treatment were paid by the National Health Insurance Corporation, and non−reimbursed items were paid by the local governments, the Korea Centers for Disease Control and Prevention, and community health centers. The entire cost of the treatment for this COVID−19 infection (excluding the cost of consumable materials) was borne by the government[103].

In fact, about KRW 9.7 million was charged for the treatment of a patient who was hospitalized for 19 days as a confirmed case of COVID−19 and was discharged after a full recovery. As all expenses related to treatment, including KRW 6 million for the negative pressure room and KRW 1 million for treatment, were paid by the government and the Health Insurance Corporation, the confirmed patient only had to pay KRW 40,000 for consumable materials such as syringes, needles, and alcohol. In addition, on April 2, 2020, the government, together with the Ministry of Health and Welfare and the National Health Insurance Corporation, discussed a healthcare institution support package to relieve financial and administrative difficulties of front−line medical institutions against COVID−19. The healthcare institution support package included health insurance support such as advance payment of medical care benefits to medical institutions, allowing them to focus on treatment for COVID−19. There was also quick budget support for establishing and operating screening station facilities, loss compensation, and loan support for healthcare institutions suffering losses in the course of responding to COVID−19. The details of the specific support plan through health insurance included salary support, treatment support, and administrative standards deferral. Salary support included the nationwide expansion of advance payment of health insurance and early payment of health insurance benefits announced by the Ministry of Health and Welfare. Supports such as the negative pressure isolation rooms for medical institutions with negative pressure isolation beds, increases in the medical fee for using intensive care units, grants for infection prevention and management, and quarantine management fees for 316 healthcare institutions qualified as national safety hospitals were provided[104].

---

103) Ilyosisa, The Irony of the Nursing Hospital "hit by COVID−19" [www.ilyosisa.co.kr]

104) Reporter Seong−soon Kwak, How Is the KRW 1.3 Trillion COVID−19 support Provided to Healthcare Institution? [www.docdocdoc.co.kr]

Other government supports to healthcare institutions' included compensation and loan support for operating screening stations and/or specialized in infectious disease hospitals. They also provided support to government−designated inpatient treatment beds operating healthcare institutions, healthcare institutions with expanded beds for critically ill patients, labor costs and protective clothing for dispatched medical staff, masks for quarantine, and mobile negative pressure equipment.

In addition, the healthcare institution support TF announced that it would consult with the government to realize the amount of advance payment for health insurance and to ease the requirements for advance payment of healthcare benefits to healthcare institutions using medical loans, while continuously coming up with specific healthcare institution support measures necessary for treatment sites. From March 23, the National Health Insurance Corporation implemented a special case of advance payment of health insurance benefit costs to healthcare institutions across the country to support the management difficulties they are experiencing due to COVID−19. Health insurance premiums for the low−income class and small business owners who are economically damaged by COVID−19 were reduced by 40 to 50%.

Although thorough management was effective in the initial stage, large−scale outbreaks occurred through religious gatherings in the Daegu, Gyeongbuk area due to the associated characteristics of COVID−19 virus that has a long incubation period as well as no initial symptoms.

However, despite the rapid spread, the large−scale diagnostic testing system in South Korea enabled rapid follow−up investigations, infection diagnosis, and quarantine measures. This was owing to the steady preparation based on the experience of the MERS coronavirus in 2015. Disclosure of movement route and time, visitors, and contacts in an attempt to transparently inform the public about the route of infection and the possibility of contact with an infected person induced voluntary quarantine activities and diagnostic tests. As there has been a conflict between individual privacy and public interest, it seems necessary to draw a social consensus on the level and scope of disclosure in the future.

A problem that arose from the beginning of the quarantine response and will keep arising in the future is the issue of immigration control for infected people. Infectious diseases are spreading worldwide and occurring with time lag. Even with thorough domestic infection control, if the inflow from overseas is not blocked, recurrence and infection will occur constantly. Considering the people who must engage in economic activities, it would be very difficult to use a lockdown policy. In South Korea, from the beginning, inbound travelers were managed with an open policy rather than a lockdown policy, but measures were taken to allow them to engage in social activities after diagnostic tests and self−quarantine for a certain period. As the global epidemic of COVID−19 continues for a long time, it is expected that strengthening quarantine measures under this open policy will have a positive impact.

When an infectious disease spreads, a temporary shortage of quarantine materials is likely to occur. In South Korea, the shortage of masks was a representative example. The mask−wearing attitude by healthcare workers and the people played an important role in quarantine activities, but there was a temporary shortage of masks. To solve this problem, the government implemented the public mask policy. This solved two problems: lowering the soaring price of masks to a price anyone can purchase (KRW 1500/sheet) and equal distribution of masks to all citizens (two per week).

In particular, the National Health Insurance played a major role. Due to the characteristics of South Korea, where all citizens were enrolled in health insurance, diagnostic tests and treatment could be received at a very low price. As the economic burden was small, most people, including the vulnerable group, could receive diagnostic tests and receive quarantine/self−treatment, which contributed greatly to preventing additional spread of the disease.

3. Directions and goals of policies to deal with emerging infectious diseases in the future

A. Need to establish the infection spread level

Blocking foreign inflows: When an outbreak of an infectious disease occurs abroad, it is necessary to prevent the outbreak by blocking the inflow of the infectious disease through immediate monitoring.

Control of domestic spreads: In the "caution" level of infection response, when the influx of an infectious disease is identified, early detection of infected persons is necessary through monitoring of major facilities and movement within the national quarantine system to prevent the spread.

All−out control of spreads: In the "severe" level of infection response, the infectious disease spreads to the local community, making it difficult to distinguish between the infected and the non−infected. The indiscriminate spread, shortage of manpower and resources could result in numerous casualties, leading to a national crisis requiring an all−out response.

Stabilization: The government should be able to manage infection routes and resource, and the number of infected and dead will decrease, allowing a certain level of normal economic activities to take place.

Normalized recovery: The end of the infectious disease is declared, the damage caused by the infectious disease is identified and compensation is made. The society will undergo the recovery process to prevent recurrence.

B. Balance between national health and economic recovery

The economic crisis is still ongoing because of the extended COVID−19 outbreak. However, quarantine activities for public health cannot be relaxed. It is not easy for economic activities and quarantine activities to coexist. The government should strive to manage the health of the people based on the principle of quarantine as a priority. In other words, it is necessary to prioritize quarantine over economic activities, and prepare financial support and policies for continuous social distancing, hand washing, and mask wearing. Nevertheless, due to changes in economic activity, efforts should be made to lower overcrowding, such as non−face−to−face services and flexible working hours. Since there is a possibility that infectious diseases will continue to occur, it is now necessary to apply the principle of quarantine as a priority in all social activities.

The V−shaped scenario represents a typical economic shock that eventually turns to growth, while the U−shaped scenario demonstrates some permanent loss of production after the initial shock. In the L−shaped scenario, substantial structural damage occurs, having a significant impact on growth.

In the past epidemics, the V−shaped scenario was observed in all cases, whereas the impact of this COVID−19 is still unknown. However, it is necessary to overcome the economic crisis by strengthening bilateral relationships and economic activities between countries through open policy rather than the lockdown. In addition, in preparation for the outbreak of the next infectious disease after the end of the COVID−19 situation, continuous investment and management of the healthcare quarantine system seems necessary.

C. Social dialog and formation of public consensus

The high−intensity quarantine response and prolonged social distancing have not only reduced the level of social and economic activities, but also have also contributed to the accumulation of stress in the people. Some citizens violated self−isolation obligations, and a crowd was gathered to enjoy the cherry blossoms without complying with strict social distancing, and some even fail to wear a mask.

The government should inform the status of the infectious disease through transparent information disclosure and gather public opinions to form a consensus for a flexible quarantine response. Setting the level of disclosing public movement of infected people, which is an ongoing issue, should be addressed based on constant communication and consensus.

D. Introduction of distancing in daily life

From April 12 to 26, the Central Disaster and Safety Management Headquarters conducted an online survey to collect public opinions on the key rules for distancing in daily life f. Distancing in daily life refers to the quarantine measures to implement social distancing in a sustainable form in preparation for prolonged COVID−19. The government proposes five key rules of distancing in daily life, including staying at home for 3 to 4 days if sick, washing hands for 30 seconds, coughing at elbows, disinfecting once a week, ventilating in the morning and evening, and maintaining a healthy physical distance (in the length of about two arms) from people. Even after the change of the daily quarantine system, physical distancing in daily life will continue, and the basic COVID−19 quarantine rules for churches, PC cafes, and private institutes will not change. The government plans to lower the level of legal and compulsory sanctions for violations of quarantine rules according to the trend of additional confirmed cases.

E. Stabilization of national mental health

After the outbreak of COVID−19, social distancing to prevent infection reduced gatherings and meetings between people, some suffered from frustration and depression. On the Internet, a new term "corona blue was created by combining the words "Corona 19" and "blue,"" which means depressed mood.

Corona blue is not a medical disease, but a psychological symptom of a social phenomenon. After the outbreak of COVID−19, emergency disaster messages and news are continuously received in association with COVID−19. The high−intensity quarantine response and prolonged social distancing have not only reduced the level of social and economic activities, but also have also contributed to the accumulation of stresss in the people.

Reference

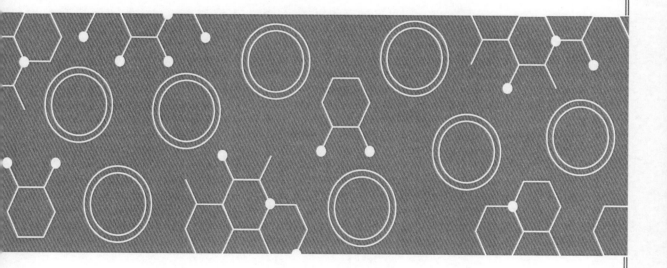

Reference

1. Bank of Korea (n.d.). National Accounts, Each Year.
2. Bok Kyu Kwon, Hyeon Cheol Kim (2009). Bioethics & Law. Seoul: Ewha Womans University Press.
3. Bora Chung (1986). The History of Dentistry Education in Korea: Universities in the Future. International Conference on the Centennial of Yonsei University, Yonsei University Press, 1986. 103.
4. Byeong Ho Choi, et al. (2007). 「Analysis data of key policy issue」. Korea Institute for Health and Social Affairs.
5. Byung−Joo Moon (2005). Industrial Relations and the Character of the Korean Welfare System: A Reinterpretation of the Industrialization Period(1963−1986). Korean Political Science Review, 39(5), 153−177.
6. Cha Heung−bong (2006). Pharmaceutical division of labor policy. Seoul: Jipmundang, 2006.
7. Choi Eun−young, et al. (1998). Prospects and Policy Challenges for Pharmaceutical Personnel. Korea Institute for Health and Social Affairs.
8. Chun Mi Kim, et al. (2012.7). Redefining the role of a health clinic and developing an implementation plan. Ministry of Health & Welfare. https://scienceon.kisti.re.kr/srch/selectPORSrchReport.do?cn=TRKO201500007029
9. Cueto, M. (2004). The origins of primary health care and selective primary health care. American journal of public health, 94(11), 1864−1874.
10. Daegu Haany University (2008). A Study on the establishment of Health Insurance Application Criteria by the Introduction of National Long−Term Care Insurance.
11. Dong−Chan Kim, On−Young Lee, Eui−Beom Jeong, and Min−Gyu Jeong (1980). 「National Transition of Endemicity of Malayan Filariasis in Inland Korea」. Report of NIH Korea. Vol. 17, 395−404. https://url.kr/bu8si2
12. Dongguk Industry Academy Cooperation (2013). A Study on the Pharmacy Manpower Project 'VISION 2030'.
13. Duk−Joon Suh, et al. (2014.7). A Study on the Present State of Medical Education in Korea: The White Book. Research Institute for Healthcare Policy.
14. Encyclopedia of Korean Culture[Website] (n.d.). National Health Insurance. http://encykorea.aks.ac.kr/Contents/Item/E0043194
15. Health Insurance Review & Assessment Service (2014). 「Establishment(close~down) of Care Facilities in 2009 ~ 2013」. https://www.hira.or.kr/bbsDummy.do?pgmid=HIRAA020002000100&brdScnBltNo=4&brdBltNo=4931
16. Health Insurance Review & Assessment Service (2015). Comprehensive Quality Report of National Health Insurance. https://www.hira.or.kr/bbsDummy.do?pgmid=HIRAA020002000100&brdScnBltNo=4&brdBltNo=6177#none
17. Health Insurance Review & Assessment Service (n.d.). Number of Provider by Year and City/Province, each year.
18. Health Right Network (n.d.). "Is the commercialization of hospitals good?". http://www.konkang21.or.kr/bbs/board.php?bo_table=free&wr_id=22614&sfl=

wr_subject&stx＝&sst＝wr_last&sod＝desc&sop＝and&page＝37

19. Healthcare Reform Committee (1997). Medical Policy Challenges (for the Advancement of the Medical Sector). Korea Institute of Health and Social Affairs.

20. Hyo Jung Lee (2012.12.27). Medipana. Civic groups 'braking' policies to promote medical privatization for an elected person, Moon.
http://medipana.com/news/news_viewer.asp?NewsNum＝100535&MainKind＝A&NewsKind＝5&vCount＝12&vKind＝1

21. In Sool Yoo (2015). Current Status and Problems of Emergency Medical Service System. Health Insurance Review & Assessment Service. p.17.

22. Jae Sik Kim, et al. (1998). 「Unification of Oriental and Western Medicine with Study on Oriental and Western Medicine」, Korean Journal of Medical History. 7(1), 47－60, 1998. https://academic.naver.com/article.naver?doc_id＝10834461

23. Jae－Won Park, Jee－Young Hong, Joon－Sup Yeom, Sung－Rae Cho, and Dae－Kyu Oh (2009). Evaluation of the Current Status of Malaria Elimination Project in the Republic of Korea and Suggestion for Improvement of Its Efficacy. Infection and Chemotherapy, 41(1), 42－53.

24. Jang Young－Sik, et al. (2010). Korea;s Population Policy Trends and Prospects. Korea Institute for Health and Social Affairs.

25. Joo Hwan Kim (2008). Historical Changes in Pharmaceutical Division Policy. Seoul: Korea Study Information.

26. Keun Lee, et al. (2007). Emergency Medical Instructor Training and Certification Report. Ministry of Health and Welfare· Gacheon University College of Medicine.

27. Kim Jung－soon (1984). Epidemiological Theory. 2000 Seoul: Shinkwang Publishing Co., Ltd.

28. Kim Young－Sook, Moon Sung－Woong, Lee Sang－Yi (2007). Health Insurance and Economic Growth. Health Insurance Forum. 6(4).
https://kmbase.medric.or.kr/Main.aspx?d＝KMBASE&i＝1138920070060040027&m＝VIEW

29. Kim Young－tak (2014). Status and Prospects of Disease in Korea.

30. Korea Centers for Disease Control and Prevention (n.d.). The collaborative network of the National Health Information Portal.
https://health.kdca.go.kr/healthinfo/biz/health/intrcnYard/nationHlthinsPortalMain.do

31. Korea Central Cancer Registry Ministry of Health and Welfare (n.d.). Cancer registration Statistics. Each Year.

32. Korea Health Industry Development Institute (2001). A study on the optimal supply of long－term care beds and specialized hospital beds.

33. Korea Health Industry Development Institute (2003). A study on the development for optimal utilization of beds.

34. Korea Health Industry Development Institute (2006). A Study on Strengthening Publicity and Operational Efficiency of Local Public Hospitals such as Local Medical Centers.

35. Korea Health Industry Development Institute (2007). Restructuring the role of public health facility with introducing Long－term Care Insurance.

36. Korea Health Industry Development Institute (2013). Handbook of Health Statistics, 2013.

37. Korea Health Industry Development Institute (2013). White paper of Health Industry 2012. Hanhak Print.
38. Korea Health Industry Development Institute (2014). A Study on the Improvement of the Effectiveness of the Bed Supply and Demand Plan.
39. Korea Health Personnel Licensing Examination Institute (n.d.). Annual Report of Korea Health Personnel Licensing Examination Institute, Each Year.
40. Korea Health Promotion (2017). Public Health Doctor System: The current status and the wat forward, Weekly Issue No. 034, 2017.
41. Korea Institute for Population and Health (1987). Research on Medical Resources and Management Systems.
42. Korea National Institute for Bioethics Policy (2012). 「Overview of relevant streams related to withdrawal of Life─sustaining treatment」. Health Law and Ethics Forum. 1(3). http://www.nibp.kr/xe/act2_2/1502
43. Korean Academy of Medical Sciences (1998). A research study on the improvement of the specialist system.
44. Korean Council for University Education (2009). Department information by University 2009, Seoul: Korean Council for University Education.
45. Korean Dental Association (1980). History of the Korean Dental Association.
46. Korean Dental Association (1987). Survey on National Dental Education.
47. Korean Dental Hygienists Association (2004). A Study on the Extension of Dental Hygienist's Work.
48. Korean Journal of Medical Education (2003). Twenty Years of The Korean Journal of Medical Education. Seoul: Korean Journal of Medical Education.
49. Korean National Tuberculosis Association (2014). Korea Health Development Corporation. Paju: Earth Culture History, 2014.
50. Korean National Tuberculosis Association (n.d.). Epidemiologic characteristics of smoking in Korea. Each Years.
51. Korean Pharmaceutical Association (2004). 『50 Years of Korean Pharmaceutical Association』.
52. Korean Red Cross (n.d.). Blood Services Statistics. Each Years.
53. Korean Society of Infectious Diseases, Korea Centers for Disease Control and Prevention, Korean Association for AIDS Prevention. (2004). HIV/AIDS guidelines.
54. Korean Statistical Information Service (n.d.). Census of Economically active population, Statistics Korea. Each Year.
55. Korean Statistical Information Service (n.d.). Family budget survey, Statistics Korea. Each Year.
56. Korean Statistical Information Service (n.d.). Household Projections. Statistics Korea.
57. Kwang─Ho Meng, et al. (1999). A Study on the Improvement of the Medical School System: The Medical Society's Position on the Recent Discussion of the Medical School System. Korean Council on Medical Education.
58. Lee In─young (2009). The Beginning and Death of Life: Ethical Debate and Legal Reality. Seoul: Samwoosa.
59. Lee Koung Kwon (2009). A study on the direction of revision of the Emergency Medical Service Act. Ministry of Health and Welfare.
60. Lee, Moo Sang, et al. (1999). A Study on the Development and Implementation of the Post─Bachelor's Degree Medical Education System Model. New Education Community Committee.

61. Ministry of Agriculture, Food and Rural Affairs. (2011). 2010/2011 Animal and Plant Quarantine Agency. https://ebook.qia.go.kr/20180306_103953/

62. Ministry of Agriculture, Food and Rural Affairs. (2014). Avian Influenza(AI) SOP. https://url.kr/wlk1y4

63. Ministry of Education & Human Resources Development (2002). 「Consistency in the Basic Plan of School of Medicine and Dental Medicine」.

64. Ministry of Health and Welfare, Korea Foundation for International Healthcare. (2014.3). 203 Modularization of Koreas Development Experience: Development of the Emergency Medical Services System.

65. Ministry of Health and Welfare, Korea Institute for Health and Social Affairs. (2019). OECD Health Statistics 2020.

66. Ministry of Health and Welfare (2000.12.11). Proposal to amend the Pharmaceutical Affairs Act through medical, contractual and orthodox agreements. Press release. http://www.mohw.go.kr/react/al/sal0301vw.jsp?PAR_MENU_ID=04&MENU_ID=0403&page=983&CONT_SEQ=19557

67. Ministry of Health and Welfare (2006). 「First Korean Medicine Development Plan (2006~2000)」.

68. Ministry of Health and Welfare (2011). 「Second Korean Medicine Development Plan(2011~2015)」.

69. Ministry of Health and Welfare (n.d.). Health and Welfare Statistical Year Book. Each Year.

70. Ministry of Health and Welfare (n.d.). Infectious Diseases Surveillance Yearbook. Each Year.

71. Ministry of Health and Welfare (n.d.). National Health Statistics. Each Year.

72. Ministry of Health and Welfare (n.d.). Patient Survey. Each Year.

73. Ministry of Health and Welfare. The Health and Welfare White Paper. Each Year. http://www.mohw.go.kr/react/jb/sjb030301ls.jsp#

74. Moon Ok−Ryun (1998). A Study on the Developmental Improvement of the Medical Security System. Ministry of Health and Social Affairs.

75. National Assembly Secretariat (2005.10.10). Minutes of the National Audit and Health and Welfare Committee Meeting. 47−48.

76. National Center for Health Statistics (2012). 「Health, United States」.

77. National Emergency Medical Center (2013). National Emergency Medical Center Statistics.

78. National Emergency Medical Center[Website] (2021.5.17). History of emergency medical center of Korea. https://www.e−gen.or.kr/nemc/emergency_medical_services_system.do?viewPage=history

79. National Health Insurance Service, Health Insurance Review & Assessment Service. (2014 3/4). 「National Health Insurance Statistical」. Number of Provider by Type and Province.

80. National Health Insurance Service. 「National Health Insurance Statistical」. Each Year.

81. National Health Insurance Service. 「National Health screening statistical yearbook」. Each Year.

82. National Institute of Health (1980). Report National Institute of Health. 17, 395−404.

83. National Institute of Health (2003). Severe Acute Respiratory Syndrome.
    http://www.mohw.go.kr/upload/viewer/skin/doc.html?fn=%25EC%2582%25AC%
    25EC%258A%25A4(SARS)%25EA%25B4%2580%25EB%25A6%25AC%25EC%25A7%
    2580%25EC%25B9%25A8(%25ED%2596%2589%25EC%25A0%2595%25EA%25B8%2
    5B0%25EA%25B4%2580)_0501.hwp&rs=/upload/viewer/result/202302/

84. National Medical Center (2010.4.2). 「National Medical Center Corporation Transition,
    New Start to National Medical Center」.
    https://www.nmc.or.kr/nmc/bbs/B0000001/view.do?nttId=5299&menuNo=2003
    93&pageIndex=26

85. OECD. (2012). 「OECD Health Care Quality Review: Korea」.

86. OECD. (n.d.). 「Health Data」, Each Year.

87. OECD. (n.d.). 「OECD Health Statistics」, Each Year.

88. Park Jiwook (2010). The Medical Assistance of Swedish Red Cross Field Hospital
    in Busan. Korean J Med Hist 19 : 189-208 June. 2010.

89. President's Council on Education Reform Commission (1995). Education reform
    measures to establish a new educational system(I).

90. President's Council on Education Reform Commission (1996). Education reform
    measures to establish a new educational system(II).

91. Seol Hee Jung, Joo Yeon Oh, Hyejin Lee, and So Young Yoon (2011). A study
    on appropriate management of the National Long−Term Insurance. Health
    Insurance Review & Assessment Service.
    https://repository.hira.or.kr/handle/2019.oak/2376

92. Sihn Kyuhwan, Seo Hong Gwan (2002). 「The Development of Private Hospital in
    Modern Korea, 1885−1960」. The Korean Society For The History Of Medicine.

93. Son Junkyu (1981). A Study on the Welfare Policy Decision Process in Korea.
    Degree thesis (Doctorate), Graduate school of Seoul National University: Political
    Science major 1981.

94. Song, Geon−Yong (2004). Improvement of the medical system. Journal of the
    Korean hospital association. 37−48.

95. Song Suk Eun (2020). A Study on Competition and Antitrust Issues in the
    Pharmaceutical Sector. Law School, Sungkyunkwan University.

96. Soon Hyung Lee, et al. (1995). A Study on the Improvement of Medical Education.
    Ministry of Education Policy Project Research Report.

97. Sorokdo National Hospital (2013). 「Newsletter of Sorokdo National Hospital」.
    http://www.sorokdo.go.kr/sorokdo/board/boardList.do?board_id=057&bn=galle
    ryList&menu_cd=03_05&depth=nn

98. Statistics Korea (2010). 2010 Population and Housing Census.

99. Statistics Korea (2015). Statistics on Changes in Korean Society in the 70th Year
    of Liberation.

100. Statistics Korea (n.d.). Annual Report of cause of death, Each Year.

101. Statistics Korea (n.d.). Annual Report, dynamic statistics of population, Each
     Year.

102. Statistics Korea (n.d.). Life table, Each Year.

103. Stjernswärd, J., Foley, K. M., & Ferris, F. D. (2007). The public health strategy
     for palliative care. Journal of pain and symptom management, 33(5), 486−493.

104. The Association of Korean Medicine (2012). 「1898~2011 History of the Association of Korean Medicine」.

105. The Board of Audit and Inspection of Korea (2011). Emergency medical services system Operation Status Audit Report.

106. The Committee for the Sixty-Year History of the Korean Economy (2010). The Korean Economy: Six Decades of Growth and Development, Ⅴ.

107. The Korean Radiological Technologists Association (1995). 30 Years of History of the Korean Radiological Technologists Association.

108. Won Joong Kim, Sang Hyuk Jung, Seung Hum Yu (1999). The Impact of the Establishment and Expansion of Medical Schools on the Social Economy. Korea Medical Association.

109. World Health Organization (1977). Report on the operations research study on basic health services in Yongin Gun Gyeonggi Province (No. KOR/HSD/001). WHO Regional Office for the Western Pacific.

110. World Health Organization (1990). Cancer pain relief and palliative care: report of a WHO expert committee [meeting held in Geneva from 3 to 10 July 1989]. World Health Organization.

111. You Bok Lee (1988). 「Contemporary History of Medicine in Korea」, Korea Academy of Medical Science. Seoul.

112. Young Il Chung (1992). Community Health and Primary Health Care, Seoul: Jigu Culture.

113. Yu Seung-Hum, et al. (1999). Diagnosis and Prescription of Korean Healthcare Problems. The Korean Society for Preventive Medicine.

114. Yu Seung-Hum, et al. (2002. 11). 21st Century Korean Health and Medical Policy Reform Direction. Korea Institute of Medicine.

115. Yu Seung-Hum (1990). Medical Policy and Management. Kirinwon.

116. Yu Seung-Hum (1991). General outline of medical insurance. Soomoonsa.

117. Yu Seung-Hum. Chang, Hoo Sun (2008). 60 Years of Korea, 60 Years of Health Care... Future Health Care Development Direction· National Academy of Medicine of Korea.

118. Yu, S. H., & Anderson, G. F. (1992). Achieving universal health insurance in Korea: a model for other developing countries?. Health Policy, 20(3), 289-299.

Acknowledgement

A special acknowledgement to the National Research Foundation of Korea(NRF) who supported the capacity building project between Yonsei and UHAS, as well as the production of this book. (No.2021H1A7A2A03098782 / Public Health Educational Capacity Development of University of Health and Allied Sciences in Ghana.)

Asian Institute for Bioethics and Health Law of Yonsei University

Asian Institute of Bioethics and Health Law of Yonsei University was established in 2002 as the first teaching researcher jointly operated by the Medical Center (medical school, dental school, nursing school, and health school) and the main school (law school, liberal arts college). Since the foundation of the institute, research has been actively conducted in various fields such as bioethics, public health, medical disputes, international health laws, and future medicine. Currently, the △ International Health Law Research Center, △ Advanced Science Research Center, △ Medical Dispute Litigation Research Center, △ Medical Ethics Center, △ Elderly and Mental Health Center are classified, approaching each field more professionally and in−depth. In addition, it continues to cooperate with overseas scholars and international organizations beyond Korea, playing a leading role in the field of "medical law ethics" in the world beyond Korea.